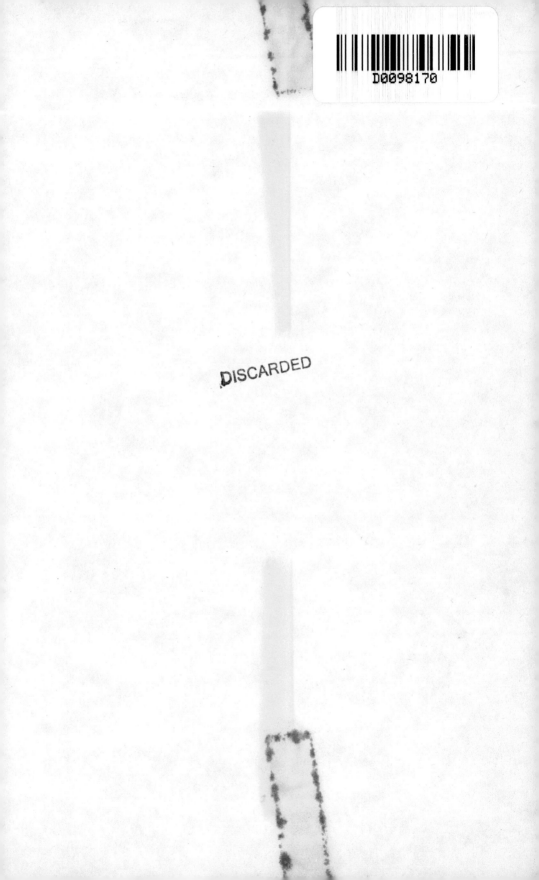

National Health Insurance and Health Resources

National Health Insurance and Health Resources

The European Experience

JAN BLANPAIN *with*

LUC DELESIE *and*
HERMAN NYS

HARVARD UNIVERSITY PRESS

Cambridge, Massachusetts, and London, England   1978

Copyright © 1978 by the President and Fellows of Harvard College
All rights reserved
Printed in the United States of America

Library of Congress Cataloging in Publication Data
Blanpain, Jan.
    National health insurance and health resources.
    Bibliography: p.
    Includes index.
    1. Medicine, State—Europe. 2. Insurance, Health
—Europe. 3. Medical care—Europe. 4. Medical
policy—Europe. I. Delesie, Luk, joint author.
II. Nys, Herman, 1951– joint author. III. Title.
[DNLM: 1. Insurance. Health—History—Europe.
2. National health programs—History—Europe.
3. State medicine—History—Europe. 4. Health
services—History—Europe. W275 GA1 B6n]
RA412.5.E85B57   362.1'094   77-25818
ISBN 0-674-26955-1

To Thomas McCarthy

fortis, ferox, et celer

Foreword

This is an important book. Through scholarly analysis and synthesis, as well as critical examination of the limited quantitative data available, Professor Jan Blanpain and his colleagues support generalizations about health services and their financing that need to be widely understood. Prepared under the auspices of the United States Department of Health, Education, and Welfare and conducted at the Institute for European Health Services in Leuven, this study should attract a wide international audience, not only among health professionals but especially among politicians responsible for health legislation. It should also be of interest to informed laymen who are concerned with the evolution of social services in Western industrialized countries.

The lessons so diligently documented and digested by the authors should guide policymakers in diverse political jurisdictions. These lessons are related less to the limited uses made of social arithmetic by legislators than to the way in which health professionals, the public, and their political leaders think about the allocation of health-care resources to meet the needs of people.

Jan Blanpain, Luc Delesie, and Herman Nys, in their scrutiny of health policies and practices in West Germany, England and Wales, France, the Netherlands, and Sweden, tease out the critical issues and identify the common factors that require appreciation if prudent investment in health care is to have a measurable impact on the health status of populations. In their brilliant series of integrating chapters on policies, the authors trace a sequence found in all the countries: early concern about providing access to physicians, then preoccupation with hospital construction, and then questions that heralded the inevitable political awakening: "Physicians and hospitals for whom and for what?" The resultant attempt to establish priorities and balance resources focused attention on health manpower and from there led to the major contemporary efforts to create comprehensive, integrated systems of health care. Again there were questions: What kinds of manpower, in what mix, do the people need? What incentives and controls should guide, or even govern, the choices? Money and its methods of transfer through a variety of insurance and other payment mechanisms are shown to be less important than reaching a calculated balance between primary or general physicians and specialists. Influence over the demand for balanced mixes of manpower is more important than controlling the supply in containing costs.

It is gradually being perceived that the response of health professionals to the distribution of problems in the population should be used to determine the mix of professionals and the mix of technology and facilities supplied to them. But achieving this goal requires that improved health information and statistical systems be assimilated by those in charge. Incentives should be built into health insurance schemes and other financing mechanisms to influence resource allocations, and priorities should be determined by the distribution of health problems and the known benefits of intervention. Such approaches are more likely to achieve reasonable public expectations than are those which disregard the political lessons so carefully documented in this book.

Health and disease reflect the human condition; they are a part of what we have been and what we are, both individually and collectively. We need to seek general understanding through vigorous application of both biomedical and behavioral sciences, and to use this understanding to improve public education, rather than attempt idiosyncratic solutions locked into parochial professional, organizational, and political notions that defy historical experiences and neglect the broader social fabric of which health and health care are only a part.

Professor Blanpain and his colleagues have deepened our level of understanding and broadened our perspectives. They have shown us that health services research and the new epidemiology are scientific tools, and that they require international development, if balanced and integrated health care arrangements, which really make a difference to the health and welfare of people, are to be created by politicians, professionals, and administrators. To all who care about these matters, I commend this book.

Kerr L. White, M.D.
Institute for Health Care Studies
United Hospital Fund of New York

Preface

In 1961 I had the privilege of visiting the Johns Hopkins University Hospital. I was on a World Health Organization fellowship, and it was my first visit to the United States. Dr. Russell Nelson, the hospital director, graciously accommodated me in the red-brick Administration Building, a proud remnant of the old hospital. It was Christmas time—I still remember vividly the nurses singing carols around the imposing statue of Christ in the central hall.

Between the whirl of Christmas parties, I got to reading Chesney's history of the Johns Hopkins Hospital and its parent university (Chesney 1958). It struck me then that John Billings, who had been appointed to direct the construction of the Johns Hopkins Hospital, had traveled to Europe in 1876 to visit the most important hospitals and to seek information. There I was, some eighty-five years later, one of many Europeans seeking to profit from America's advances in medical care and hospital management. At that time I could not visualize that the pendulum would swing back yet again one day, and that I would be highly involved in the subsequent shift of interest.

America is again interested in learning from European experience, in particular in the domain of the organization and financing of health care. Distinguished American scholars like Renée Fox, Kerr White, Odin Anderson, and others, increasingly include Europe in their studies and publications on health care. Study visits to Europe are frequently undertaken by American government envoys, congressional committees, and the like. An interesting aspect of this development has been that Europeans themselves have responded to the American interest with a greater alertness about the health care situation in other countries.

During an extended stay in 1971 as visiting scientist at the National Center for Health Services Research and Development of the U.S. Department of Health, Education, and Welfare, I became acutely aware of the American interest in European health services. On my return to Leuven University, this exposure helped to strengthen a tradition of research on health care in the European Economic Community and led to the creation in 1972 of the Institute for European Health Services Research. The publication that follows results from a study made at the institute in 1975–1976 under contract (HRA-230-75-0108) with the Division of Legislation, Health Resources Administration, U.S. Department of Health, Education, and Welfare. I was privileged to be joined in the study by dedicated associates, first by Luc Delesie and Herman Nys, co-authors of this publication, and second by Jan Debie and Johan Lievens, who shared the burden of data collection. Count Gibson of Stanford University Medical School, who during the time of the study joined the staff of the Leuven Institute, addressed himself to the problems of the health consumer and brought a valuable dimension to our undertaking.

Without the help and good will of a great many individuals and agencies, this study could not have been completed. It is hardly possible to name them all, yet I feel I should mention some for their special efforts. John Moscato, director of the Division of Legislation and project officer, deserves special gratitude for his sound guidance and effective assistance in bridging transatlantic distances. Anne-Marie Denef, our administrative assistant, and Malinda Coleman, our editorial assistant, provided unique support, meeting expectations that many authors allow themselves but only a happy few see realized. Among my colleagues at Leuven University, I wish to thank in particular Lou Groot and Pol Quaethoven for their valuable comments.

Special thanks are extended to our advisors in the survey countries. They read draft texts of the chapters on their respective countries and discussed the work at special meetings with the research team. The national institutions that were hosts for these meetings deserve special appreciation. For the Netherlands, assistance was given by Professor J. De Vreeze, president of the National Hospital

Council; Dr. J. H. Baaij, head of the Division of Policy Development, Ministry of Public Health and Environmental Hygiene; Professor A. Querido, emeritus professor of social medicine, University of Amsterdam; L. L. Marselis, secretary-general of the Sickness Fund Council; and A. Polderman, secretary of the National Sickness Funds Organization. For France, the advisors were Dr. Bridgman, inspector-general for social affairs, Ministry of Health and Social Welfare; Professor Péquignot, professor of clinical medicine at the Paris V University; the late Dr. Rösch, research associate at CREDOC; Mr. Michel, honorary director of the National Federation of Offices of Social Security; and Ms. Sirel, advisor for the plan, Office of the Prime Minister. The German advisors included Dr. U. Geissler, Federal Ministry for Labor and Social Affairs; Dr. J. Lauterbacher, associate director of the German Hospital Association; Dr. S. Eichhorn, trustee of the German Hospital Institute; Dr. R. Schicke, director of the Task Force on Hospital Research and Organization, Medical School of Hanover; Dr. N. Henke, of the Institute for Social Legislation at the Ruhr University at Bochum; and Dr. P. Swertz, of the German Hospital Institute. Participating for Sweden were Professor B. Rexed, director-general, National Board of Health and Welfare; Professor R. Berfenstam, professor of social medicine, University of Uppsala; G. Högberg, director at SPRI; H. Wilhelmsson, head of the Planning Division, National Board of Health and Welfare; and E. Jonsson, research associate at SPRI. The participants for England and Wales were Sir George Godber, former chief medical officer, Department of Health and Social Security; G. McLachlan, secretary of the Nuffield Provincial Hospitals Trust; Professor B. Abel-Smith, professor at the London School of Economics; and Sir John Revans, formerly regional medical officer, Wessex Regional Health Authority.

Professor Duncan Neuhauser of Harvard University reviewed our manuscript and offered incisive comments and valuable suggestions, for which I will remain most grateful. Dr. William Bennett, editor for science and medicine of the Harvard University Press, coached us in the intricate procedure of bringing the manuscript into final print. Working with him was a real pleasure, and I will never forget his trust and confidence. A special word of thanks goes to Christiane Dekeyser, Arlette Lemmens, Monique Wouters, and Mia Veuchelen, who typed and retyped the manuscript. The omissions and defaults

that readers will undoubtedly detect in this book are my sole responsibility. This provides part of the motivation to continue the work,
which, who knows, may lead to yet another book.

Jan Blanpain, M.D.
Leuven

Contents

National Health Insurance
and Health Resources

1 | Introduction

As of February 1976 eighteen national health insurance bills had been introduced in the Ninety-fourth Congress of the United States of America. Six of these bills were identical to bills introduced during earlier legislatures, eight bills were modified versions of earlier bills, and four were new proposals. This intense legislative activity reflects an ongoing debate in the United States on the desirability, feasibility, scope, and technicalities of national health insurance. Furthermore, most of these bills were preoccupied with health resources and with measures to improve the delivery of care (Waldman 1976).

The preoccupation with health resources and health care delivery is not new; rather, it is a measure of prolonged concern over inadequacies in the American health care system, which is perceived in an ambivalent way: a mixture of pride and frustration, of appreciation and disenchantment. *Doing Better and Feeling Worse,* the paradoxical title of a 1977 report on health in the United States prepared under the auspices of Nelson Rockefeller's Commission on Critical Choices for Americans, epitomizes this ambivalence. In his introduction to the report, John Knowles, president of the Rockefeller Foundation, writes that "The American people have clearly come to expect much from medicine, especially in recent years, but they have matched these rapidly rising expectations with rising anxieties over the cost, quality and accessibility of health services" (American Academy of Arts and Sciences 1977, p. 4). National health insurance is thus being considered as a possible solution for this problem and as a potential vehicle for major change in the current ways of organizing and delivering health care. One way of exploring this possibility is by examining how other countries use health insurance and how

their health insurance schemes relate to the more general development of health resources. In other words, how did European governments develop health resources in support of their national
health programs? This is the main question to which we address our-
selves in this study of five countries. In an attempt to answer it, we
analyze European experiences with health resource development in
light of the emerging policies for national health insurance in the
United States.

Most of the leading American proposals for national health insurance include specific measures to remedy maldistribution of services,
discontinuity in care, cost inflation, and uneven quality (American
Hospital Association 1974). This preoccupation with effectiveness
and efficiency in the delivery of health care is different from the
more restricted and specific role envisioned for national health insurance by most of the European countries. In Europe, the predom-
inant reason for the introduction of national health insurance has
been to provide economic security and to enhance social justice. For
example, in the United Kingdom, the National Health Insurance
Act of 1911 was basically an attempt by Lloyd George to prevent
poverty caused by sickness. It therefore focused mainly on restoring
the wage earner's financial self-reliance, by permitting him to overcome income losses due to sickness and by restoring his capacity to
earn money. Dependents were excluded from this program, which
was entitled "national health insurance" only just before its introduction, instead of "national income insurance," a more appropriate
term.

The public debate over national health insurance has taken different forms in Europe and the United States primarily because in
Europe national health insurance was introduced before or shortly
after the beginning of this century: 1883 in Germany, 1911 in the
United Kingdom, 1928 in France, and so on. At that time, the effectiveness and efficiency of the production and delivery of services
were largely overshadowed, if considered at all, by the basic need to
insure against the economic threat of disease and disability. The
United States first considered the introduction of national health insurance at the same time as Europe, at the turn of this century, in
reaction to forces similar to those in Europe: industrialization; urbanization; employment policies that threatened unemployment;
work-related injuries and diseases; and the likelihood of economic
catastrophe for families in case of illness, where the natural support

of the extended family of an agrarian society was no longer available. In contrast to Europe, however, in America the movement towards social security programs was implemented only through selected income security programs. Although national health insurance had been a lively issue in the United States before World War I and was revived again and again, health insurance developed mainly on a voluntary basis, through, on the one hand commercial insurance programs, and, on the other, Blue Cross-Blue Shield plans; the latter were initiated and to some extent controlled by the main providers of health care: hospitals and physicians. Only in 1965 was a partial form of national health insurance introduced through Medicare and Medicaid. The mixture of approaches that had been allowed to develop resulted in an extremely complex pattern of financing of health care in the United States. The employed are predominantly covered by contributions to either nonprofit voluntary insurance (Blue Cross and Blue Shield) or to commercial insurance. The aged have a combination of compulsory insurance for hospital care financed from tax revenue (Part A of Medicare) and a voluntary insurance for physician services (Part B of Medicare). The latter is financed by individual contributions and federal subsidy. The Medicaid program uses local, state, and federal tax revenue towards the medical needs of the indigent and medically indigent. Special groups in the population, such as veterans, merchant seaman, and Indians, receive direct provision of services in special facilities. This complexity in the financing of health care has been, together with other crucial aspects of today's health care scene, a compounding factor in the prevailing conviction that the United States health industry urgently needs integration, coordination, planning, and regulation.

Tying change to financing is a logical reflex, particularly when the opportunity is as great as it is in the United States, where nearly all parties involved seem to welcome, for different reasons, the idea of national health insurance. As major purchasers of health insurance, industry and management see an opportunity to transfer part of the financing responsibility from themselves to general taxation. Labor wants to improve its bargaining position for direct pay increases by diminishing the pressure of health insurance contributions on the payroll. Hospitals and physicians see in national health insurance a mechanism to guarantee income and adequate compensation for services. Insurance agencies hope to stabilize and strengthen their position by undertaking the actual administration of such a program (Batistella 1971, p. 20). Thus, nearly all groups concerned realize the need for measures to improve the delivery of health care and they support those measures. In fact, the whole debate on national health insurance in the United States has centered on the degree of financial and health protection to be provided to the citizenry, and the appropriate methods for reorganizing the health care system, rather than on the question of whether to do either.

Long experience with voluntary health insurance, and a decade of coping with limited forms of compulsory health insurance for selected groups, have brought the lesson home to nearly everyone that mechanisms which merely raise money and redistribute it to health care providers in return for services given under defined conditions (coverage, eligibility, co-payment, restrictions in time and kind, for example) are, regardless of their actuarial sophistication, not sufficient to guarantee that everyone in need of health care will receive it in an efficient and effective way. Furthermore, the current economic situation seems to preclude a massive expansion of federal budgetary intervention in American health financing. As President Ford remarked in his State of the Union address on January 19, 1976, "We cannot realistically afford federally dictated national health insurance providing full coverage for all 215 million Americans." In view of this, some, like H. Somers, have suggested abandoning the strategy that seeks to link measures for reorganization of the health care system to the enactment of national health insurance (Somers 1972).

In fact, while the national health insurance debate continues without resolution, rationalization of the health care system and of health resources development is already being pursued. A number of actions taken by the Congress since 1972 indicate a determination to come to grips with some of the health care system's basic problems, as identified in the national health insurance proposals. The Social Security Act Amendments of 1972 (P.L. 92-603) introduced professional standards review organizations. Their role is to assess the necessity and quality of medical care delivered under programs supported by federal money (Decker and Bonner 1973). Prepaid practice plans providing a comprehensive range of medical services with emphasis on preventive action were given support through the 1973 Health Maintenance Organization Act (P.L. 93-222) (Dorsey 1975). Major health planning legislation was enacted in 1974 (P.L.

93-641), providing a nationwide network of health systems agencies. These are designated to serve distinct health services areas and are mandated to plan and develop health resources within state health plans and following national health planning guidelines (Anderson and Robins 1976). Under P.L. 94-484, the Health Professions Educational Assistance Act of 1976, nearly $2.7 billion was authorized for health manpower development within terms and conditions seeking to redirect the supply, the functional mix and the spatial distribution of health manpower (Department of Health, Education, and Welfare 1976). And, as suggested earlier, the national health insurance bills themselves contain specific measures reflecting several avenues along which the health care system could be rationalized. The Ullman bill and the Staggers bill stress planning and organization of a comprehensive, well-distributed delivery system. Assurance of quality care is emphasized in the Young bill and the Fannin bill. Cost containment through less costly alternatives to hospital care is pursued in the Staggers bill and in the Corman-Kennedy bill which also provides for resources development through grant mechanisms (Waldman 1976).

The common denominator of these measures is health resources development, and the U.S. Department of Health, Education, and Welfare is fundamentally concerned with health resources development in support of national health insurance. While our study was initiated to provide background for the formulation of health insurance, health care, and health resource development in the United States, it also attempts to offer European scholars and policymakers a unique historical perspective on resources development within neighboring systems.

Conceptual Framework

Successive policies for health resources development have evolved throughout the long history of national health insurance in the five European countries we studied: England and Wales, the Federal Republic of Germany, France, the Netherlands, and Sweden. Our analysis and comparison focuses on the nature, content, origin, and interdependence of those policies, on the issues that guided their development, and on the forces that shaped their format and impact. Such an analysis holds valuable lessons for any country trying to improve its health care system.

The key concepts in the study are, on the one hand, "national health insurance" and, on the other hand, "health resources development," both of which need to be clearly defined at the outset. Unfortunately, the term "national health insurance" is a loose and inexact expression, understood differently in the five countries under study and in the United States. In the five European countries, funds from general revenues have been added to the funds raised by payroll deductions and individual contributions in order to pay for health care. National government involvement varies from country to country, and has varied within individual countries, from the requirements that certain categories of workers purchase private insurance, at one extreme, to the provision of the entire health service itself, at the other. In the United States, meanwhile, the term "national health insurance" is used to refer to national programs which, through a combination of contributory and general revenue financing, together with government regulation of the delivery of health care, aim to make comprehensive health care universally accessible, at a certain standard of quality and within certain cost limits.

Certain archetypes typify the different roles played by national governments in financing health care and in providing health care. A gradient of increasing government involvement is reflected in the archetypal methods of financing. Under the type with minimal involvement the working population is required to seek private insurance, with the government purchasing such insurance on behalf of the indigent. A next type is direct national insurance financed by contributions earmarked for health services only. In the ultimate type, national insurance is paid for by general treasury funds, an important alternative because compulsory payroll deductions are a regressive form of taxation. The transfer of a major portion of health care financing to general revenues represents a significant step in income redistribution. Three typical roles, also reflecting a gradient of involvement, are played by the government in providing health care. The first role is largely an indirect one whereby the government seeks to regulate the availability of services, controls the costs and the quality of the care provided, and acts as mediator when complaints or conflict arise. Acting as contractor of services is a more involved role of the government. The ultimate stage is the direct provision of services by government agents and facilities.

Thus, because of the different meanings applied to it, use of the term "national health insurance" as a frame of reference for the study of health resources development could lead to the comparison of different entities, and therefore to confusion. To make this frame of reference comparable, therefore, and to contrast prevalent national health insurance proposals in the United States with comparable European realities, the term "national health insurance" must be replaced with the broader concept of a "national health program."

National Health Program

In this study, the common frame of reference to which health resources development will be related is the national health program. This term refers to the aggregate of existing and intended national arrangements regarding the financing and (or) provision of health care that have emanated from the national legislative bodies or from the national government. The aggregate of existing and intended arrangements includes the whole spectrum of the legislative and government actions for the development of a national health program: policy proposals, action proposals, legislative proposals, bills, acts, regulations, plans, and actual implementation.

Health Resources Development

Three categories of health resources can be distinguished: human resources, physical resources, and information resources. During the course of this study, a second type of classification emerged. This second classification, in three levels of increasing organizational complexity, reveals a growing capacity for developing a comprehensive health care system, and coming to grips with the crucial issue of relating health resources development to the system's needs.

First level, or basic, resources are the basic inputs of every health care process. The health care process consists basically of interactions between health care consumers and health care providers, both depending on specific knowledge and on specific material provisions. Basic health resources fall into the three categories mentioned earlier: human resources, physical resources, and information resources.

1. Human resources include health care providers (physicians, dentists, pharmacists, nurses, and allied health professionals) and health care consumers.
2. Physical resources include health care buildings, health care equipment, drugs and vaccines, and biomedical research labs.

3. Information resources include biomedical knowledge and health behavior knowledge.

It can be argued that these basic health resources are interdependent. For example, biomedical knowledge can be considered either as an input to the education of a health care provider, or as an output of the research activities of that health care provider. Nevertheless, these basic health resources do exist as separate entities, and result from clearly definable activities: education, research, construction, and production, for example. Simple combinations of basic health resources—such as a generalist with elementary instruments and a limited medical library—permit the provision of health care. More complex combinations of basic health resources result in organizations and institutions that provide for identity, continuity, and specialization of the activity to be undertaken. These combinations involve a second level of health resources.

Second level, or managerial, resources are required to plan, organize, and administer basic resources into organizations and institutions that meet some health needs under conditions of quality assurance, effectiveness, and efficiency. Again, managerial resources include human resources, physical resources, and information resources.

1. Human resources include hospital administrators, health care planners, health services administrators, health statisticians, and health services researchers.
2. Physical resources include computer hardware, training schools, and health services research institutes.
3. Information resources include health status information (information on the health status and health needs of defined populations—for example, household health surveys), health resources information (information systems on health resources—for example, health manpower statistics), health care activity information (information on utilization, costs, outputs or outcomes of health care activities—for example, hospital discharge abstracts information systems), and health research information (information on health research activity—for example, medical literature retrieval systems).

It can be argued that these managerial resources are also interdependent; for example, health information systems involve data as well as computer software technology to manage the data. Simple combinations of second level or managerial resources provide specific health care-related organizations or institutions with a common goal. For example, a hospital bookkeeping system, together with some managerial expertise, will allow for some hospital budgeting.

More complex combinations of managerial resources result in the third level of resources: multi-organizational, or health system, resources. Combinations of basic resources and managerial resources are always associated with some organizational scheme or program; for example, a group practice involves some primary physicians and some managerial expertise to streamline their activities, and a school health program involves special kinds of basic resources, such as a school-aged consumer group, allied health professionals, and management by some type of administration. Health system resources are required to plan, organize, and administer basic resources and managerial resources within multi-organizations or supra-organizations to meet comprehensive health needs under conditions of quality control, effectiveness, and efficiency. Health systems resources are of recent origin. The human resources, physical resources, and information resources at this third level are:

1. Human resources: health care system scientists, medical research policy makers or coordinators (for example, special ministers), regional health care planners, and coordinating bodies.
2. Information resources: macro model of a given health care system, detailed national health accounts, and national utilization statistics.
3. The physical resources: the same as for managerial resources, though definitely more complex.

Health resources development is usually understood as the quantitative expansion of given categories of health resources, such as increasing the supply of doctors or raising the number of hospital beds. However, the term "development" also has qualitative connotations, such as "improvement" or "innovation." Integrating existing health services, creating a new type of health worker, improving the health consciousness of the population, and providing for consultation of the population on regional health care plans are all examples of qualitative development.

This study addresses itself to both quantitative and qualitative development. But, besides broadening the conventional concept of "development" in this positive way, the study also considers "development in reverse," as indicated by policies and proposals, some of recent date, aimed at slowing the growth of given resources or reducing the supply of certain resources. We also acknowledge that governments depend greatly on a range of nongovernmental institutions for health resources development; educational and research institutions, institutions in various industries involved in health care (pharmacy, technology, construction, and, recently, management consulting), and various voluntary, semipublic, or public regulating institutions.

With respect to health resources development, then, governments basically have four options. First, health resources development can be left to market forces. A second option is to affect existing institutionalized developers, for example, by providing financial support, by reorganizing programs, and by providing new incentives. A third, more fundamental, option is the creation by government of new institutionalized developers. The last option is to influence health resources directly, for example, by importing doctors from abroad, curbing export of doctors, importing drugs or advanced technology, and providing financial incentives. Regardless of the option chosen, health resources development is influenced by different pressure groups, such as organized providers, organized labor, reimbursement groups, universities, and consumer groups.

Method of Approach

The initial step in undertaking a study of national health insurance and health resources development is to select the countries appropriate for examination. In the current case, England and Wales, France, the Federal Republic of Germany, the Netherlands, and Sweden were selected by the United States Department of Health, Education, and Welfare, the study's sponsor. We were ambivalent about this choice of countries. On the one hand, the number of countries involved, and particularly the need to cope with five different languages in a limited time, presented a formidable challenge. On the other hand, the choice provided a rich variety of different geographic, demographic, and socioeconomic conditions, of different historical developments and different health care systems. We were particularly pleased that American interest in European experiences had widened from the traditional scholarly preference for the United Kingdom and Sweden to include nations on the European mainland. The sponsor also provided a method of approach by outlining three sets of questions to be answered by the study: questions pertinent not only to the options confronting American policymakers but also to the interests of a wider audience.

The first set of questions pertained to the *recognition* of the need for resources development. In each country, what were the problems confronting the national health program at a given moment? Did the public authorities recognize the need for development at that time? Did they recognize this need for all types of resources or was the attention concentrated on some specific types?

The second set of questions focused on the *objectives, scope,* and *process* of resources development. What were the objectives? Were they intended to stimulate short-term improvement, or were they formulated as part of a general strategy for the health care delivery system? Was this part of social and economic planning? Were these objectives the result of a democratic process? What mechanisms and pressure groups influenced their formulation? Was it influenced by certain events or circumstances? Were the objectives attained? Were there any unexpected side effects?

The final set of questions focused on the central issue of this study: the *role of government* in health resources development. Was special health resources legislation enacted? What administrative mechanisms were mandated to carry out health resources development? Can market forces be relied upon to adjust to the needs of a national health program, or should government intervene in providing for resource development? If government is made responsible for resources development, what levels of government should be responsible? Also, what elements of health resources, manpower, physical resources, and other factors should be expected to require special assistance? Do different approaches to health resources development present advantages or disadvantages?

In attempting to answer these sets of questions and to identify health resources development policies that supported the national health program in each country, we used two chronological approaches. One approach was to look at the national health program throughout its evolution, to see whether the legislators had provided for, or intended to provide for, resources development. The framework of health resources and resources development, as described above, was applied in this examination. A second approach was to look at those health resources which tend to be better documented, such as hospitals and physicians, and to trace the development of each, the policies that had shaped this development, and the relationship of the resource to the national health program. Given the breadth of material and timespan to be covered (with national sickness insurance having been introduced in Germany in the nineteenth century), certain limits had to be established. For example, the development of one specific resource could have been studied in great detail within the context of the evolving national health program; the findings of such a limited but detailed approach could then lead to conclusions about the full spectrum of resource development. However, the sponsor required information on a range of health resources. This requirement had two potential pitfalls: first, that by trying to survey every possible resource within sensible limits of research resources, we would come up with results at a level of meaningless superficiality; second, that by attempting to cover the whole history of the different national health programs, we would present conclusions swamped in massive detail. So, for feasibility and efficiency, two major restrictions were established. The first was to focus on crucial episodes in the history of each national health program, such as the introduction of a compulsory insurance scheme or major changes that occurred or were considered for the program. These crucial episodes were used as vantage points from which questions were addressed. The second restriction was to refrain from examining certain health resources, in particular, drugs and medical research. Medical research in Europe has recently been investigated by a joint effort of the Ciba Foundation and the Wellcome Trust (Excerpta Medica 1973). Many European comparative studies on drugs are currently being sponsored by the World Health Organization and are being performed at the Council of Europe and also, in particular, by S. Sandier and colleagues at CREDOC in Paris (Siderius 1975).

The method of inquiry followed three major steps. Prepared with detailed background information on the country, study team members visited each country, to identify, in consultation with leading national scholars and government officials, those critical episodes in the history of their national health programs that should be used as entry points for the study. Second, the research team prepared a draft text for each country, on the basis of the conceptual framework and available documented evidence. Finally, in a second visit to each country, the draft text and the conceptual framework were subjected to a group discussion, in which the research team was joined again by national scholars and top officials of the national health program. Confronted in a group with a conceptual framework that had been applied to their own system, the experts were able to react in a focused way, to provide valuable refinements where the draft contained wrong assumptions and factual errors, and to check on each other's inputs. Having witnessed these mutual checks during the group discussions, the research team was reinforced in their conviction that the traditional method of addressing questions separately to a number of individuals often results in conflicting information and in analyses that are rejected after publication, as incomplete and inaccurate, by reviewers in the particular countries.

The Countries

Although the Federal Republic of Germany, France, England and Wales, the Netherlands, and Sweden are all parliamentary democracies located in Western Europe, these five countries are significantly different in geography and demography, in their constitutional and administrative systems, and in the basic principles of their health care systems as they exist today. An overview of these differences provides an essential background to a comparative evaluation of their differing approaches to health resources development.

Geography and Demography

Table 1 summarizes geographic and demographic data that are significant for the health resources development of the five countries. Some of the differences shown in this table result in marked differences in approach to health care delivery. For example, the relatively low population density in Sweden makes the distribution of health care providers far more problematic than it is in a country like the Netherlands. Nevertheless, all five countries share two major demographic trends that are extremely important in the design of health care delivery systems: the concentration of the population in large urban areas, and an increasing average age, caused partly by a diminishing birth rate. The urban concentration of population is most dramatic in Sweden: between 1950 and 1970, 82.5 percent of the country's population increase took place in the Stockholm and

Gothenburg regions, and in 1975, 81.3 percent of the population lived in urban areas (The Swedish Institute 1975). In less densely populated parts of Sweden, the problems of health care delivery are quite severe: while the average density is 18 per km², the concentration in urban areas (229 per km², in Stockholm) is offset by extremely low densities in the most rural areas (3 per km² in Norbotten, the most northern county of Sweden).

All the other countries display a similar, though less pronounced, tendency toward urban concentration of population. For example, 46 percent of the Dutch population lives within the Randstad, the triangular area in the west of the Netherlands that encompasses three major cities: Amsterdam, Rotterdam, and The Hague (Ministry of Public Health 1974). In England and Wales in 1972, 80 percent of the total population lived in urban areas, with 20 percent in the Greater London area (*Britain 1974*). Similar patterns exist in France and the Federal Republic of Germany.

As for population aging, Table 1 shows that at present Sweden is confronted with the human, financial, and political problems associated with an aging population more immediately than the other four countries are. But declining birth rates in all five countries indicate that it is only a matter of time before this trend will begin to exert its pressure everywhere.

Constitutional and Administrative Systems

As parliamentary democracies, each of the five countries has a government that consists of a head of state and a parliament; the supreme power lies with the people, as represented by members of parliament. However, there are marked variations among the five countries in the details of this system, notably in the relative balance of power between the head of state and the parliament, and between the parliament and the government ministries, since there has been a general shift in power in most countries from the legislative to the executive bodies.

In three countries, England and Wales, the Netherlands, and Sweden, the head of state is a hereditary monarch. Since 1975, when the Swedish constitution was reformed, the Swedish monarch has no longer performed any political functions; his responsibilities are limited to ceremonial duties. The privileges of the British and Dutch monarchs have also diminished over time, but they both still have certain political responsibilities, such as signing governmental decisions and selecting prime ministers. Nevertheless, their real power or influence is not easy to measure. While the head of state in both France and the Federal Republic of Germany is a president, the German president's status is roughly that of a ceremonial monarch; the chancellor heads the government and defines the country's political orientation. Only the French president can claim to exercise significant power, a variation that is due to de Gaulle's 1958 constitutional reform, in which the president gained considerable powers at the expense of the French parliament. President Giscard d'Estaing's dismissal of Prime Minister Chirac, in October 1976, demonstrated the extent of this presidential privilege.

In all of the countries but Sweden, parliament consists of two chambers, in which members of the first chamber are not directly elected to their positions (in some cases, as in England and Wales, seats in the first chamber are hereditary), while members of the second chamber are directly elected. Sweden abolished its first parliamentary chamber in 1971, on the grounds that it was undemocratic, and a similar trend appears to be emerging in some of the other countries, through a limitation of the first chamber's constitutional responsibilities.

Broadly speaking, the parliamentary legislative process falls into three stages. In the first stage, a bill is drafted and introduced into one of the chambers. In the second stage, a standing or ad hoc parliamentary committee discusses the bill extensively. Finally, in the third stage, the bill is debated and passed or defeated. Where there are two chambers, a bill passed in one chamber must go through the same three stages in the other before it becomes law. Although, constitutionally, members of parliament in all countries have the right to initiate legislation, there is a common trend towards minimizing parliament's legislative functions and increasing ministerial or other involvement in the origination of bills. As mentioned earlier, in France the constitutional reforms of 1958 restricted parliament's legislative functions to certain subjects; and the federal structure of the Federal Republic of Germany requires in many cases that federal parliamentary power give way to state parliaments. Even in the other three countries, parliamentary legislation tends to take the form of a general framework only, to be filled in with statutory regulations by government. The formulation of this framework is further affected by the considerable involvement of royal commissions, whose members are drawn from outside the government and even from outside parliament.

In all five countries, advisory committees can intervene in the legislative process: departmental committees (composed of top civil servants), standing or ad hoc parliamentary committees, and a variety of other committees representing specific interest groups, known in general as "the fifth power." The involvement of these different committees sometimes slows down the legislative process, but it has the advantage of permitting all sides to be heard and of allowing a concensus ultimately to evolve.

The ministries holding executive responsibilities for health care matters vary considerably from country to country in their range of responsibilities, both functionally and in the geographic decentralization of the executive powers. In terms of the functions actually assumed by health ministries, England and Wales represent one extreme, where the administration of health services has been almost entirely unified with that of social services within the Department of Health and Social Security (following the 1973 reorganization of the British National Health Service, the DHSS also took over the School Health Service from the Department of Education and Science). A similar situation exists in both France and the Netherlands. In France, the ministries of Health and Social Security were merged a few years ago. In the Netherlands, the Ministry of Public Health and Environmental Hygiene administers both the health care delivery system and health insurance benefits (the benefits in kind, not the cash benefits). In contrast, in the Federal Republic of Germany, responsibility for administering health care services and executing relevant legislation is widely dispersed among different ministries: the Federal Ministry of Youth, Family, and Health (health care); the Federal Ministry of Labor and Social Affairs (health insurance); the Federal Ministry of Economic Affairs; and so on.

Finally, the Swedish administrative system presents a unique pattern, in which administration is divided between two types of authorities: on the one hand, the different ministries (such as the Ministry of Health and Social Services), each with a small staff responsible for formulating policy and regulating administrative agencies, and on the other hand, central administrative boards (such as the National Social Insurance Board and the National Board of Health and Welfare). These boards, which can be considered as special-purpose agencies, employ the bulk of Sweden's civil servants, and are headed by powerful directors-general. Although the boards are autonomous, and independent from their corresponding ministries, the directors-general have in recent years become increasingly integrated within the relevant ministries, with the result that the authority of the ministries is increasing. Thus, the National Board of Health and Welfare receives its instructions and directives directly from the government.

Apart from their variations in functional responsibility, the health ministries in the different countries vary in the degree to which they delegate responsibilities to smaller units, such as regions and municipalities. As administrative and executive tasks are delegated downward, a ministry's own responsibilities become more indirect: setting frameworks, establishing guidelines, and so on. In Sweden, at one end of the spectrum, government is highly decentralized towards the middle and local levels. At the middle level, twenty-three countries and three county boroughs are governed by elected county councils, which are responsible for a number of services, mainly in the health care field, including general hospitals, district medical officers, mental hospitals, and dental care. They levy their own taxes. At the local level, 278 communes provide a number of facilities, including housing, water supply, and basic education (The Swedish Institute 1974).

The provision and administration of public services in England and Wales has traditionally been characterized by a unique balance of local autonomy and central control. However, since the end of World War II, central government has taken many functions away from local government, and the administration of health services at regional and local level has been separated from the administration of other regional and local authority services. In April 1974, Regional Health Authorities (fourteen in England, one in Wales) and Area Health Authorities (ninety in England, eight in Wales) were established to assume health care responsibilities at the regional and area levels. Because of the concept of "co-terminosity," the Area Health Authorities correspond geographically to the local authorities. The basic operational unit within these authorities is the district (*Britain 1974*).

In France, despite important recent efforts to decentralize towards the regions, which are now the most important health care settings, the state remains unitary and centralized. The lower administrative levels continue to have only minor responsibilities in health care matters.

The Netherlands are in a process of transition with respect to decentralization. A reorganization of regional and local government is under way (the provinces are to be more than doubled in number), and a bill was introduced in October 1976 to involve the regional and local authorities in the administration of the health care system in a decision-making capacity (Ministerie Volksgezondheid 1976).

Finally, because of its federal structure, the Federal Republic of Germany presents an exceptional pattern. As mentioned above, each of its eleven states has legislative powers that it can exercise independently of the federal legislature. Each state also has a separate health administration, headed by a Ministry of Labor, Health, and Social Affairs. However, at local and regional level, the situation is largely similar to that in France and the Netherlands.

Basic Principles of Health Care Systems

While an examination of the history and present form of the health care systems of the five countries reveals that they differ greatly, some common trends emerge when we consider whether the governments intervene directly in the provision or financing of health care or whether they act indirectly, with health insurance playing a significant role in financing. In general, the countries fall into two groups. In the first group, England and Wales and Sweden, government intervention is direct, and private health insurance plays a marginal role. In the second group, the other three countries, government intervention is much less significant, and health insurance schemes cover most health care costs, though in ways that vary from country to country.

In England, then, about 90 percent of the costs of the National Health Service are paid for from general revenue. Hospitals are publicly owned, and specialists are either part-time or full-time salaried hospital staff. General practitioners, most of whom own or rent their own offices, are paid a yearly fee per patient treated, determined through negotiations between their representatives and the government. The number of state-owned health centers, however, is growing. Dentists are paid on a fee-for-service basis. Prescribed drugs are provided at a small charge, and pharmacists are paid according to a schedule negotiated with the government.

The Swedish system is similarly characterized by publicly owned hospitals, although they are organized by the county councils. The importance of hospital care in Sweden is reflected by the high ratio of hospital beds to population (see Table 1). Inpatient care is provided by salaried physicians. Ambulatory care is provided in hospital-based clinics, also by district doctors salaried by the county councils, by salaried physicians employed by enterprises and corporations, or by private physicians whose fees are paid through social insurance. National health insurance covers health care costs only marginally, the main burden being carried by county income taxes. The patient pays an insignificant portion of the actual cost at the time of illness.

While health insurance schemes are much more significant in meeting health care cost in France, the Federal Republic of Germany, and the Netherlands, quite different schemes operate in each country. In France, health care is provided: (1) by private general practitioners or specialists, of whom an increasing number are working in group practice; (2) in dispensaries managed by municipalities, sickness funds, trade unions, or nonprofit associations; and (3) in public (65 percent) and private hospitals. Sixty-three percent of these health care services are paid for by public health insurance, 27 percent by the patients themselves, 5 percent by the central and local authorities, and another 5 percent by private health insurance. French public health insurance is provided through a complicated group of "legal schemes": the general scheme, the agricultural scheme, special schemes (for civil servants, miners, railway personnel, and other groups), and the voluntary scheme, which covers the 2 percent of the population not compulsorily insured by another scheme. Apart from these legal schemes, there are the complementary schemes, entirely private, which are important because they provide insurance against risks covered only partly, or not at all, by the legal schemes.

In the Federal Republic of Germany, about 55 percent of the hospitals are publicly owned. An interesting characteristic of the German system is that hospital care is restricted to inpatients. Except for teaching-hospital outpatient departments, ambulatory care is provided outside the hospitals, by physicians in office practice. More than 90 percent of the German population is compulsorily insured by the sickness funds. The remaining 10 percent is insured mainly through private sickness insurance. Except for private patients, no direct financial exchange takes place between the patient and his physician or hospital. Free practicing physicians are paid through the sickness funds affiliated physicians groups, and hospitals on the basis of per diem claims.

The Dutch national health program is a largely voluntary system, in which health care is provided mainly through voluntary nonprofit institutions and programs. Nearly 75 percent of Dutch hospital beds are under voluntary ownership. Physician services are available from community-based general practitioners and from specialists, the latter increasingly using hospital-based outpatient facilities. Health care is paid for through a social insurance scheme that combines catastrophic risks insurance for the entire population with compulsory sickness-fund insurance for workers under a given income level (70 percent of the population). Other categories of workers can insure themselves voluntarily with the sickness funds, and yet other categories are insured with private insurance companies. General practitioners are paid according to the number of their patients, and they control referral to specialists and hospitals. Specialists are paid on a fee-for-service basis, while hospitals are reimbursed on the basis of negotiated per diem costs.

I | The Countries

2 | Federal Republic of Germany

The world's first social security system was originated in Germany in 1883, when Bismarck made sickness insurance compulsory for part of the working population (Gesetzliche Krankenversicherung 1883). Since then, the fundamental principles underlying this scheme have never been changed, although the program has gradually been extended to cover about 90 percent of the German population. During the first half century of the scheme's existence, great efforts were made to institutionalize the relationship between physicians and the sickness funds, resulting, over the years, in several amendments to the 1883 Act. Eventually, these amendments culminated in 1931 in the so-called July Agreement between organized medicine and the sickness funds. Germany came out of World War II with most of its hospitals destroyed. Because of reconstruction and renewal measures, however, only one decade after the war Germany's supply of hospital beds was already considered excessive, and it was unevenly distributed over the country. This situation, together with the financial difficulties facing the hospitals, led to the 1972 Hospital Act (Gesetz zur wirtschaftlichen Sicherung Krankenhaüser 1972).

1883: A World Premiere

Already in 1838, official regulations existed in Prussia, backbone of what was to become the German Empire, requiring employers to make specific contributions towards the costs of health care for their workers. Mutual benefit societies and welfare institutions had also been organized by the wage earners themselves, and provided sickness benefits, disability and funeral benefits, and pensions to widows. At first the mutual benefit societies and welfare organizations were voluntary, but a Prussian law of 1854 made membership in such societies compulsory for miners. In the same year, Prussian districts were given a legislative mandate to enforce the organization of benefit societies and to determine contributions in case the local authorities failed to do so (Sigerist 1960, p. 122). The example set by Prussia was followed by other states as they became part of the German Empire.

Bismarck's introduction of compulsory health insurance into the German Empire in 1883 was the result of a unique combination of political and socioeconomic forces. After a series of abortive attempts, the German Empire had been founded in 1871, with William I, king of Prussia, becoming emperor of Germany, and Bismarck becoming chancellor. The newly created empire was rapidly confronted with an economic crisis, mainly resulting from the 1870–1871 war against France. The crisis peaked in 1874 and raised the specter of substantial social unrest, bringing back memories of the 1848 revolution. Confronted with this crisis, Bismarck saw that social legislation was necessary to deflect a development threatening the empire (Sigerist 1960, p. 121). Being a Prussian aristocrat, he reacted paternalistically (Kulp and Schreiber 1971, p. 19). His party, the Conservative party, identified itself with the state, and viewed the state's role, and therefore its own role, as one of "protecting the underprivileged." Basically, Bismarck intended to alleviate poverty, and to some extent, to remedy economic inequality; but in doing so he also wanted to preserve the existing political power structure, which implied a continuation of existing political inequality (Stump 1973, p. 207). Thus, he tried to use social insurance as a political weapon, a tool of social and political control (Rimlinger 1971, p. 130).

An important codeterminant of the social security legislation was pressure arising from the Social Democratic party, a revolutionary party that represented the industrial workers. Although in 1871 it had won only one seat to the Reichstag, by 1877 it occupied twelve seats. Bismarck tried to stop its growth with social legislation. In contrast to what happened later in other countries, at that time the German trade unions were mainly interested in the immediate improvement of working and living conditions, and they were not so attracted to the Social Democratic party's proposed long-term reforms of German society. So Bismarck responded to the trade unions' expectations and, in fact, exploited trade union opposition to the Social Democratic party and its program (Sigerist 1960, p. 125).

Bismarck's original idea was to provide a centralized and unified insurance system that would protect all economically weak groups, including agricultural workers. It was to be financed by contributions from employers and employees, and by government subsidies. Organized corporations would replace the occupational groups in administering the insurance system (Sigerist 1960, p. 128). The most important compromise Bismarck had to make was to implement the program through the existing network of sickness benefit societies (Schellenberg 1968, p. 6). Minimum benefits were set and annual reports were required. The consequence was a large group of powerful local funds that could outbid each other through variation in benefits beyond the minimum set by law, resulting in a disturbing lack of uniformity and a complicated administrative machinery.

The Sickness Insurance Act was promulgated on June 15, 1883, and came into operation on December 1, 1884. It was part of a set of acts introducing several social insurance programs: accident insurance (1884) and old age and disability insurance (1889).

The Sickness Insurance Act of 1883 required that industrial workers and other categories of wage earners up to a certain income limit be insured through existing funds or through the newly created communal funds. Some funds provided coverage for dependents on a voluntary basis. Cash payments in case of working incapacity were the most important benefit at the time. Medical care was considered secondary. This explains why even today in Germany sickness insurance lies within the authority of the Ministry of Labor and Social Affairs rather than the Ministry of Youth, Family, and Health, which is responsible for health policy.

Under the 1883 Act, the insured received physician services, medication, eyeglasses, bandages, and hospital treatment when necessary; all were free at the time of service. The compulsory scheme was financed two-thirds by workers' contributions and one-third by employers' contributions. The existing funds were governed by representatives of the employers and employees in proportion to their contributions. The communal funds were governed by locally elected representatives.

Silence of the Profession

The medical profession in Germany had already, in the 1850s, expressed its views on a state system of health services and concurrent resource development. The profession had then argued that a reform of medical services was needed because of health hazards due to the industrial revolution and the concomitant urbanization. They postulated that health care should be a basic right for workers; the state's role was to ensure that the human resources needed for a strong industrialized and defensible state remain healthy (Sigerist 1960, p. 123). In 1883 however, proposals for a state system of health care no longer aroused support and commitment. When it was established, compulsory sickness insurance meant an extension of coverage to all wage earners and an increase in the amount of money earmarked for physician services. The profession was remarkably silent. History would not repeat itself in this respect.

The July 31, 1931, Agreement

Fifty Years of Confrontation

In 1931 the German government ratified an agreement between the medical profession and the sickness funds (Lynch and Raphael 1963, p. 37). This ratification was the culmination of decades of conflict and confrontation between the powerful sickness funds and the physicians. It created a national arrangement, which is still in operation today, for the financing and provision of physician services. In the years since, many measures have been taken that have related, directly and indirectly, to this agreement of July 31, 1931, and which have determined present-day relations between physicians, health insurance companies, and the government.

What were the problems leading to the 1931 agreement? Certain amendments of the 1883 Act, amendments that were introduced on April 10, 1892, authorized the sickness funds to limit the number of physicians allowed to practice for insurance patients and to determine which physicians were to be employed by the sickness funds; the sickness funds were also empowered to determine the amount set aside for professional remuneration (Lynch and Raphael 1963, p. 45). In practice, these amendments led to individual contracts between physicians and sickness funds. The gradual increase in the number of insured workers created a situation in which the funds enjoyed a very strong bargaining position. They used this position to enforce low remuneration, which more and more doctors considered unacceptable. Physicians also objected to the fact that patients were limited in their choice of physician to those enlisted by their sickness fund. From 1892 on, these issues, the physicians' access to sickness fund practice and the patients' freedom-of-choice, dominated the discussions between sickness funds and the medical profession.

The physicians realized that they needed to organize themselves to counteract the increasing power of the sickness funds, which had themselves started to form into a national union (Lynch and Raphael 1963, p. 38). In 1900, Dr. Hartmann in Leipzig created, through the League of German Physicians, what was to become the powerful and militant Hartmannbund (Albrecht 1975, p. 140). Organized medicine entered into open conflict with the sickness funds (Lynch and Raphael 1963, p. 40). Local strikes occurred, for example, in Cologne in 1909, where the sickness funds tried to break the strike by importing physicians (Schadewaldt, Grzonka, and Lenz 1975, p. 47). The opposition of organized medicine polarized around the 1911 National Insurance Act. This act introduced a substantial rise in the income limit for compulsory sickness insurance and extended its field of application to include servants and agricultural workers, for example. Although it made written contracts between doctors and sickness funds compulsory and subject to supervision by the National Insurance Office, the act was perceived by the medical profession as a further erosion of their economic position and their basic principles: freedom of choice for both patient and doctor, fee-for-service payment, and a limited role for sickness funds. The Hartmannbund prepared for a general national strike, to start on January 1, 1914. The government made attempts to reconcile the two parties, and at the eleventh hour, on December 23, 1913, an agreement mediated by medical school faculty was signed in Berlin (Schadewaldt, Grzonka, and Lenz 1975, p. 69). The agreement included the following points (Naschold 1967, p. 57):

1. Practice size was introduced and set at one physician per 1,350 insured members, or per 1,000 members when family members were also covered on a voluntary basis.
2. A register was introduced to record physicians interested in holding an appointment with a sickness fund.

3. Appointments for insurance practice were to be made by a committee composed equally of physician representatives and fund representatives.
4. A contract committee, also equally composed, had to approve any individual contract between a physician and a sickness fund.
5. Arbitration services were made available by the government.

The issue of free choice was left open and eventually resulted in a wide range of differing local arrangements.

The 1913 Berlin agreement was signed for a ten-year period. Shortly after it was signed, World War I broke out. The consequences of the war upset all the elements in the equation. The postwar economic crisis drove the strained relationship between the medical profession and the sickness funds into a new confrontation. Doctors were competing for insurance practice, preinflation contracts were still being honored (including terms of remuneration) by the sickness funds, and the financial situation of the sickness funds was becoming precarious. These developments overwhelmed the voluntary arbitration mechanisms provided in the 1913 agreement (Albrecht 1975, p. 143). When, in October 1923, the ten-year period of the 1913 agreement came to an end, an emergency decree (Notverordnung 1923) was passed to transform the agreement into an act that would provide an official arbitration mechanism, standards for contracts, rules for remuneration of physicians, and protective measures against excessive claims. Nevertheless, the medical profession went on strike shortly after the emergency decree was passed, and the strike lasted nearly three months. It came to an end in February 1924, when the Ministry of Labor prevailed; their interpretation was that the 1923 decree had only made into law what had already been agreed upon in 1913 (Albrecht 1975, p. 180). Germany just started to recover after the currency reform of 1924 when the world depression hit with full force. From conflict to conflict, both parties—the profession and the sickness funds—inched toward a collective agreement in which sickness funds would give up some control on the number of physicians and the physicians would be enrolled in sickness fund practice in return for control on medical utilization, to be done, however, by the medical profession. As a result of this long period of conflict, moreover, the relationship between the doctors and the sickness funds became highly institutionalized, through articulate regional and national organizations and through arbitration mechanisms.

Scope and Content of the Agreement of July 31, 1931

The important elements of the 1931 agreement were (Lynch and Raphael 1963, p. 46):

1. A standard contract was to be worked out by the funds' and physicians' national associations.
2. Signing of the contract and the negotiations on relevant clauses was to be left to the regional branches of the fund associations and physician organizations.
3. Contract committees composed of representatives from both parties were to supervise the implementation of the contracts. They were also mandated to act as a first level of arbitration.
4. A physician utilization control mechanism was to be implemented. The physicians working for sickness fund patients would be organized into sickness funds affiliated physician groups. These sickness funds affiliated physician groups would designate physician committees with the specific task of supervising medical utilization within the sickness funds. The sickness funds themselves were allowed to delegate some of their own physicians to these committees. The sickness funds took upon themselves the task of collecting all necessary statistics, which were then given to the committees for evaluation.

The 1931 agreement meant a victory for the physicians in Germany. The preceding measures on social insurance had all concentrated on the sickness funds. They had created a powerful national machine that was in fact directing health insurance and health care development in Germany. But, in 1931, the physicians' fight to gain national recognition was won. Previously they had been dealt with individually; now, group recognition at national level was achieved.

From 1931, the physicians determined, by and large, their own destiny. Although a physicians' control mechanism was included in the 1931 agreement, this mechanism was rather unsophisticated: moreover, it was totally in the physicians' hands. The sickness funds never pushed to improve its effectiveness. During the first and second decades after the agreement they would have been unable to do so if they had wanted to. Indeed, the victory of the National Socialists in the 1933 elections resulted in the toning down of the powerful national apparatus that the sickness funds had built up. On the other hand, the National Socialists strengthened the role and influence of the medical profession. The political programs during the period stressed health as a national priority—health at any price. The responsibility for attaining this goal was felt to lie with the medical profession, which was given the means it needed to implement this mandate. A central national body, which all physicians had to join, was constituted for this purpose.

The utilization control mechanism anticipated by the 1931 agreement, however limited it may have been, thus had no chance at all during the National Socialist period. Indeed, it was politically unthinkable that an area of such prime national interest should be subject to limitations or controls at all. The shift in power from the sickness funds to the physicians' organizations permitted the physicians to assume autonomous control over the health care sector.

Health Insurance after World War II

Germany, at the end of the war, had a strongly organized medical corps that had achieved a high social status. The sickness funds machinery had completely deteriorated. Moreover, there were over 1,500 funds, organized in seven main groups: general local sickness funds, land sickness funds, factory sickness funds, trade association sickness funds, seamen's sickness funds, miners' sickness funds, and mutual benefit funds. The first four groups were made up of local funds; the last three were national funds. The negotiations between the sickness funds and physicians demonstrated the funds' weak position: physicians were represented in these negotiations by the stable sickness-funds affiliated physician groups, while the different sickness funds' representatives were constantly changing. This situation was inherited from the Nazi period and no attempts were made after the war to alter it.

The Allied Powers had done everything possible, however, to dissolve the Third Reich, as reflected in the 1949 Basic Law, which established the Federal Republic of Germany. (The Basic Law is not called a constitution in order to avoid a legal affirmation of the separation between East and West.) The Basic Law reveals a clear shift in power from the central government (the Bund) to the states. In health care matters, it means that the states are responsible for health affairs and health insurance, insofar as the Basic Law does not confer specific legislative powers to the federation, or insofar as the federation does not use its legislative powers.

The federal government used its basic legislative prerogatives for the first time in 1955 to amend the National Insurance Act of 1911. This amendment—the so-called Federal RVO Amendment of 1955—affirmed the provisions of the 1931 agreement, including the rules that allowed the sickness funds to limit the number of sickness funds affiliated physicians in relation to the number of subscribers (one physician to six hundred subscribers in 1931, and one to five hundred in 1955). According to different informed sources, the 1955 amendment resulted in the sickness funds affiliated physician groups acquiring a still more powerful position. By 1955, however, different sickness fund groups had tried to reactivate the utilization control machinery of the 1931 agreement. They replaced the traditional lump sum payment system for physician services with a fee-for-service scheme. By 1962, the fee-for-service payment system was generally in force, but by then the motive to exercise greater control had totally ebbed away.

The dominant issue in the evolution of the German health insurance scheme since 1960 has not been how to update the control mechanism of 1931, but how to regulate the physicians' fee structure. In 1965, the Federal Minister of Youth, Family, and Health promulgated the first Tariff Structure for Physicians, applicable to fees for private as well as sickness funds patients. However, because the funds and the sickness funds affiliated physician groups negotiated fees independently from the ministry's tariff structure, the federal government lacked instruments to control the increase of fees. Therefore, the 1965 act was subsequently amended to incorporate the fee negotiations mechanism used by the sickness funds and the profession. However, this proposal failed, and even now the federal government has no effective control over physician fees. Recent government attempts to control fees, with the object of containing costs, encountered go-slow action by the medical profession in February 1977 (*Der Spiegel* 1977).

The Hospital Finance Act, 1972

On August 31, 1954, the federal minister of economic affairs, using his authority in matters of price control, promulgated instructions to stabilize the hospital bed reimbursement rates. As in other industrialized countries, hospital costs in Germany had begun to rise steeply. If these costs were to be refunded by the sickness funds, the insured would have to pay much higher contributions. Because of these financial pressures, the federal government limited the charges and per diem claims that hospitals could present to sickness funds. The excess costs were to be covered by contributions of the hospital owners, public authorities, or private sponsors, or, in last resort, by hospital profits (Eichhorn 1973, p. 88).

One of the main sources of the increasing deficits were the depreciation rates that had been applied by the Federal government. These depreciation rates, for long-, middle- and short-term investment, were not realistic. Moreover, as the state subsidies were insufficient to pay for investment expenses, the municipalities and the counties were asked to increase their share of the hospital costs. In 1966, an official federal government inquiry estimated the accumulated hospital deficits at two billion Deutsche marks ($800 million). The federal price regulations had made an organized financing system totally impossible, since, in calculating the hospital per diem rates, they had considered principally the financial capacity of the sickness funds to reimburse these costs.

Apart from these financial troubles, there was a complete lack of hospital planning. Hospitals had developed in an isolated and uncoordinated way. Each state responded differently to its hospital legislation responsibilities. Most states preferred to finance new hospitals, but they did not close down the old ones. As a result, the Federal Republic of Germany found itself confronted with a large number of small hospitals and an extremely uneven distribution of beds and specialties among the states (Eichhorn 1973, p. 83). This problem was subsequently compounded by an oversupply of beds following postwar reconstruction. This expansion also led to a shortage in hospital personnel.

Because of this uncoordinated post–World War II hospital development, the divergent approaches pursued by the states in short-term solutions to their hospital problems, and the growing hospital deficits, federal intervention could hardly be postponed any longer (Herder-Dorneich 1970). However, any federal action was blocked by the constitutional division of legal powers between the federation and the states, in which only the states were empowered to intervene in the financing and organization of health care. Thus, if the federal government wanted to solve hospital problems, it needed to change the constitution. However, such a change required a two-thirds majority, and neither of the two biggest parties, the Christian-Democrats or the Social Democrats, could force the issue on their own. Finally, the two parties formed a national coalition in 1966, which made cooperative action feasible. On May 12, 1969, this coalition government finally acquired the constitutional authority to legislate the economic situation of the hospitals. After consulting all parties interested, the federal government (by that time a coalition of Social-Democrats and Liberals) put forward a proposal on hospital financing and bed rate regulation on December 17, 1970. After the third session in the Bundestag, the bill was sent to the Bundesrat. On March 24, 1972, the Bundesrat rejected the proposal and decided to call for the formation of the Intervention Committee, an ad hoc committee provided for in the constitution in cases of such dispute. The Intervention Committee reached a compromise on May 1, 1972. Basically, it entailed separating facility-starting and maintenance costs from actual investment costs, with the former being charged to consumers rather than being paid for by regulated subsidies. The act was passed on June 29, 1972, by a vote of 249 for, 2 against, and 245 abstaining.

Content of the 1972 Hospital Finance Act

The 1972 act regulates not only the financing of hospitals but also the scope and conditions of regional hospital planning in relation to population needs. The Federal government intends to use the grant-in-aid mechanism contained in the act to correct the widespread and uncoordinated growth of hospitals. Further, the act aims at keeping hospital rates within socially acceptable limits.

The act uses a broad definition of a hospital: "any institution in which there is provision of medical and nursing care for illness, pain or injury, and where the latter are diagnosed, cared or alleviated, or where provision is made for maternity aid, and to which a patient may be admitted or treated," but excludes hospitals under federal responsibility, prison hospitals, police hospitals, and hospitals belonging to life insurance funds or to accident insurance funds (Eichhorn 1973, p. 89). At present, it is unclear whether ambulatory care facilities are covered by the act.

To provide economic support for hospitals, the act provides for investment subsidies. Subsidies can be given either to meet debts or to recover depreciation costs. Grants-in-aid are possible to build new hospitals, to buy or lease equipment for existing hospitals, to meet financial charges for loans, and, in exceptional cases, to cover starting costs. The federal government distributes the financial aid among the states on the basis of approved hospital plans (state and federal). The states divide the financial support among the individual hospital projects, subject to their conformity with the state hospital plan. Existing hospitals are eligible for state support towards investment financing only if they are included in the state hospital plan. Hospitals with less than a hundred beds are not eligible unless they are explicitly included in the state plan. Grants used for purposes not fitting the state hospital plan can be reclaimed. To control the hospital per diem rates, the 1972 act specifies the conditions under which the federal hospital tariffs can be determined for all hospitals, including those not eligible for investment support. In accordance with this provision of the act, per diem price regulations for all hospitals were issued (Verordnung 1973).

Positions of Interested Parties

During the fifties, some of the sickness funds wanted the federation to intervene in the financing of hospitals. They proposed that all hospital investment costs should be met by the federal government. This proposal became part of the Social Democrats' political program. The Christian Democrats and the states were against federal funding, while the municipalities and the counties were in favor of it. In 1966, the Federal Association of Local Sickness Funds stated that, "in the interest of the public," federal long-term hospital planning was indispensable (Schlauss, p. 9).

The physicians were less involved. Private practice physicians were not at all affected by these problems of hospital financing. Hospital physicians were not sufficiently organized to form a political pressure group. The two most important physician associations did favor a basic legislative change, because they were convinced that it would improve the hospitals, and hence the hospital physicians' situation. The German Hospital Association published its own proposal on August 4, 1970, and tried to present it as an alternative to the government bill (Deutsche Krankenhaus Gesellschaft 1970). The Association also published an official comment on the federal government's proposal (Deutsche Krankenhaus Gesellschaft 1971). Its criticism was, first, that the proposal did not guarantee optimal and sufficient medical care and, second, that the hospitals would have to pay for their financial improvement by sacrificing their independence. Similar criticisms were made by other parties. A more general comment was that the bill (and consequently the act) paid no attention to other problems such as the need to reduce inpatient care, the need for coordination among hospitals, and the role of the hospitals within the total health care delivery system.

In 1974, the German Hospital Association and the major sickness fund associations made a joint proposal on the integration of ambulatory and inpatient care. The general practitioners disapproved the proposal because they believed it was an attempt by the hospitals to annex all ambulatory care services. The German Hospital Association and the sickness fund associations responded to these criticisms by proposing an experimental model. The "Advisory Report on Test Case Experiments with respect to pre-inpatient diagnosis and post-inpatients treatment," published on July 15, 1975, contained this model. It aimed at need-responsive health care involving efficient, less expensive hospitals and acceptable hospital prices. It also called for shorter in-patient stays and for improved hospital utilization without jeopardizing medical effectiveness. Two final criticisms of the 1972 act have been that the federal government has not given specific directives for planning and, according to the sickness funds, that the act has caused an unusual increase of hospital costs.

Human Resources

Physicians

As in the other countries under study, governmental intervention in Germany first focused on the training of physicians. An act of 1869 made physicians' training uniform and required a proficiency test for admission to the profession. These regulations were changed on May 28, 1901, to specify what students could be admitted to what kind of schools. In the same year an internship period was added to the curriculum, lengthening the period of medical education from four and a half to six years. Over the following years the duration of the medical curriculum continued to change regularly (Rachold 1967, p. 3).

The medical curriculum also received some attention from the National Socialists. On July 7, 1939, a new medical registration regulation was enacted (Rachold 1967, p. 5). It made internship obligatory for all students and required that they work under the direct supervision and instruction of a director or physician in an approved hospital. The training itself involved six months (later four) of nursing practice, six weeks of factory work or farm work, and six months of work as a nursing aide, as well as obligatory lectures and clinical activities. For obvious reasons, after the war the 1939 registration regulation proved impossible to maintain.

Thus, the medical curriculum was one of the first areas of physician development restructured by the federal government after the Second World War. In 1949 the German Medical Faculty Congress developed a proposal for new appointment regulations. One of the main problems dealt with was the internship period. Should it take place during or after the period of formal study? The preclinical curriculum and final examination also posed problems. Although the constitution reserved the matter for the state ministries of education, the federal government nevertheless enacted, unchallenged, on September 15, 1953, a new compromise appointment regulation (Rachold 1967, p. 11), effective from April 1, 1954, that was intended to do away with the legacy of World War II. Internship was lengthened to two years, clinical training was shortened, and a package of natural science courses was added to the medical curriculum. As a result, medical education was lengthened from six and a half to seven and a half years.

Because of the increase in medical course work, the intensification of bedside teaching, and the need for small group teaching, the amount of instruction and the number of examination subjects increased. In the following years, other changes were occasionally warranted. An amendment to the constitution, enacted on May 12, 1969, gave the federal government formal power to start planning in cooperation with the states for national education. From this amendment new government actions emerged with respect to physician education. New accreditation regulations became effective in October 1970, regulating the pattern of the medical curriculum in considerable detail—for instance, by listing the practical courses required of every student as well as the minimum number of hours per course (Approbationsordnung 1970).

The second area of governmental influence on physician development, in addition to its influence on the medical curriculum, involved the organization and regulation of medical practice and its managerial elements. The 1955 amendment of the 1911 National Insurance Act touched on different aspects of the organization of medical practice by separating hospital and nonhospital medical practice completely and by consolidating the 1931 agreement with a further reduction of the ratio of physician to insured to 1:500. In 1965, the federal minister of youth, family, and health promulgated the first tariff structure for physicians, establishing a fee-for-service scheme applicable to private as well as sickness fund practices. The size of individual fees in sickness fund practices was, however, to be discussed at state (or regional) level between physicians and funds. The scheme was organized according to medical specialty, and the different medical services subject to fund reimbursement were identified in some detail. Although the act stated only one fee figure, it also noted that an individual medical act could be differentiated according to its complexity, that a physician could take into account the patient's financial means, and that the physician could exceed the stipulated fees.

From 1965 until 1971, physicians and funds adhered to the fee-for-service system specified in the act, with, however, two important, legally correct, adjustments: First, the multiplication factor (which, according to the act, could vary from one to six to differentiate for complexity of service, financial status of the patient, and so forth) was agreed upon by both parties each year, and increased annually; and second, additional fees were also agreed upon. Both adjustments resulted in a wide range of actual fees, varying according to state, type of physician, and type of service. In other words, the federal act of 1965 did not achieve control over physician remuneration or over the volume of physician services.

In 1972, the federal government tried to amend its 1965 tariff structure for physicians. The proposed amendment was far from drastic. It maintained the notions of fee-for-service and of a fee range and granted the physician his individual right to increase fees unilaterally. Nevertheless, the proposal failed because the states blocked it, apparently because of physician lobbying. Meanwhile, physician fees kept rising. In January 1977, the government introduced a bill aiming at linking the increase in physician fees with the increase in the gross national product. This would have diminished the yearly increase in fees by about 50 percent. The physicians reacted angrily and introduced a go-slow (*Der Spiegel* 1977).

While these developments were taking place in physician practice, with the federal government intervening to little avail, another problem emerged from a different source: the widely varied conditions in which German physicians had to practice medicine. In Germany, major differences in socioeconomic status, population density, and geography separate the cities and the rural areas, the richer and the poorer states, and the industrialized and the heavily agricultural states. Working conditions for physicians are far from homogeneous, and these variations have undoubtedly resulted in considerable unevenness in the distribution of physicians. Different states and insurance funds have used different incentives to attract physicians. Free housing, for instance, has been commonly used to attract physicians to rural areas. In 1975 the federal government introduced a proposal aimed at a fair distribution of sickness funds affiliated physicians and a strengthening of suburban and rural medical practice in areas underprovided with medical care (Bundesministerium 1975, 7:3336). The Bundesrat questioned the federal government's proposal. It considered the regulations insufficient, first because they did not address the question of what was to be done if planning according to need were not carried out, and, second, because the concept of "underprovided with medical care" was difficult to define in legal terms. The Bundesrat proposed a more far-reaching bill.

The federal government's proposal was also criticized by the Christian Democrats as being too extreme and leading toward socialization of the health care system. Paradoxically, the Christian Socialist party, the Christian Democrats' sister party, which is heavily represented in Bavaria, considered the federal proposal too mild and favored the Bundesrat proposal, which had been introduced by the Bavarian minister of social affairs (Pirkl) and was attractive particularly because of very limited availability of medical care in Bavaria. The State Ministers' Conference, the local communities and the labor unions, however, strongly favored the federal proposal. Similarly, the general practitioners favored it, primarily because it was not as far-reaching as the alternative put forward by the Bundesrat. Eventually, the federal proposal was approved by parliament in 1976, although it had been amended somewhat. The unamended bill itself contained four levels of intervention (Bundesministerium 1975, 7:3336). In the first place the sickness funds, together with the sickness funds affiliated physician groups, were to develop plans for the availability of primary care physicians in the different regions. If the mere publication of these plans proved insufficient to generate response for an improved distribution, according to criteria to be determined by July 1977, the second level of intervention gave organized medicine the opportunity to redirect the maldistribution. In case of failure, then upper limits would be established, barring primary care practitioners from moving into "over-doctored" areas. Finally, if the situation remained unsatisfactory, the sickness funds would be allowed to bring about a solution by attracting physicians to underserved areas with benefits such as free housing, free medical equipment, and loans.

The most striking difference between the proposed bill and the act that was passed is that the latter did not contain the fourth level, although the first three stages were retained, more or less (Gesetz Weiterentwicklung 1976). The sickness funds affiliated physician groups have to develop plans for each individual state to assure the availability of primary care for sickness fund patients. These plans have to be designed in conjunction with the sickness funds associations, after consulting the state authorities and in accordance with federal guidelines. The plans have to be publicized. If the physicians and sickness funds cannot agree either party can call for the intervention of a joint committee in which physicians and funds are represented. The sickness funds affiliated physician groups must take every measure, financial or otherwise, to assure, improve, or advance the availability of primary care.

The federal guidelines have to indicate which requirements are to be fulfilled to assure a reasonable availability of primary health care for sickness funds patients. At the state level, these guidelines then can be used to check whether an "underserved" situation exists or is likely. The authority responsible for this decision is the state committee of physicians and sickness funds. If this committee concludes that an area is "underserved," it can limit the free establishment of physicians in neighboring areas. But, before doing this, the committee has to permit the sickness funds affiliated physician groups to take their own measures to ease the situation, although within a specified period. If they have no results, a decision can be taken to make establishment dependent on a permit. This permit indicates the conditions and the period during which the physician will be allowed to practice in the area.

Finally, the German government is involved in determining the supply of physicians. On this subject, a remarkable fact must be remembered: after the introduction of the Sickness Insurance Act in 1883, the number of physicians increased much more rapidly in

Germany than in countries without compulsory sickness insurance, although a direct causal effect has not been established. From 1889 to 1898, the German population increased by 11.5 percent, while the number of physicians increased by 56.2 percent. In the United Kingdom, from 1891 to 1901, the population increased by 12.8 percent while the number of physicians increased by 16.0 percent; in the United States, from 1890 to 1900, similar figures were 20.7 percent and 25.9 percent (Sigerist 1960, p. 137).

Both World Wars also led to increases in enrollment in German medical schools by those seeking exemption from the draft. Furthermore, after World War II there was an influx of East German doctors, one of the reasons underlying the building of the Berlin wall. At present, entrance to German medical schools is very strictly limited: of 29,134 applicants in 1976, only 5,042 were admitted. The applicants are not selected by the medical schools, but by a central screening institution, located at Dortmund and established in 1972 by a common decision of the states. Selection is based primarily upon examination results. In January 1977, the Constitutional Court criticized this selection mechanism as being at odds with the constitutionally guaranteed freedom of education. The court stated that a selection system would be constitutional only (1) if all applicants had a chance to be selected through a lottery system instead of by examination results, which automatically eliminate the "less good"; and (2) if the medical schools functioned at full capacity, which is not presently the case.

Other Health Personnel

Germany's first regulation on nursing and paramedical personnel was enacted on September 28, 1938 (Gesetz Ordnung Krankenpflege 1938). Through this regulation, the Ministry of the Interior received the authority to develop the different health professional groups, using uniform directives. After the Second World War, however, many states themselves took the initiative to regulate nursing and paramedical personnel development (Niedersachsen in 1947; Schleswig-Holstein in 1947; Bremen in 1949). The Federal government retook the responsibility in 1957 because some uniformity had proven to be necessary. Their new regulation of the nursing profession was, however, limited to practice approbation only (Gesetz Ausübing Berufes des Krankenschwester 1957). Germany has an acute shortage of nursing personnel and is therefore actively developing nursing manpower. All parties—the hospitals, the professional associations, the states, and the federal government—are involved in this effort, and many nursing personnel studies have been undertaken.

The practice conditions of other health personnel groups have been regulated by the federal government along similar lines (Gerfeldt 1959, p. 126): medical-technical assistants in 1921, 1929, 1940, and 1958 (the last regulation provides federally uniform practices); sickness gymnasts and masseurs in 1958 (before this date, the different states had their own regulations); and midwives in 1938, when legal qualifications for the profession of "midwife" were established (Hebammergesetz 1938). Some new types of health service professionals, primarily management oriented, have also developed recently. Two universities, Munich and Düsseldorf, have founded a Public Health Service Academy. No other efforts to develop health managers have yet been identified, except the German Hospital Institute's continuing education programs.

Health Consumers

Health insurance is administered through more than 1,500 local autonomous sickness funds. The local funds are concerned chiefly with negotiating fee schedules with physician groups and have played virtually no role in processing patient complaints. Thus, consumer representation has been vitiated by a lack of power and by an inability to catalyze changes in the system. Likewise, there is no evidence that the public representatives on the boards of nonprofit, private hospitals have been able to represent the consumer. In any event, these hospitals contain only one-third of the country's total hospital beds. The pattern of consumer representation appears similarly bleak for the future. The role for consumers in health care planning has been negligible so far. But two organizations have made efforts to represent consumers. First is the Arbeitsgemeinschaft der Verbraucher (AGV); this organization attempts to assess the quality and suitability of various products sold to the public. Its resources are meager and its monthly publication slim. In the health area, it has supported efforts to improve food purity and to protect the public against participation in drug trials without consumer consent, but it has not so far attempted to investigate medical care itself.

A recent and potentially exceptional organization is the German Patients' Protection Association, founded towards the end of 1974. It lists some of its goals as follows:

a public accountability of the German medical care system

a review of university expenditures for the health professions, with justification for numbers of faculty and student body

a demand that medical organizations be less self-interested and concern themselves more with the quality of care

a drive toward "demythification" of the health profession and a more equal relationship between physician and patient

For Germany, these proposals are novel, and it is too early to predict how widely this organization will be supported. So far the traditional consumer representatives in Germany have not been very effective, and newer organizations are scarce.

Physical Resources

Hospitals

As early as the fourth century, hospitals were founded in Germany by religious orders (Adams 1973, p. 19). At the end of the Middle Ages, city authorities stepped in to participate in the administration of many hospitals. In 1794 Prussia put all hospitals under the protection and the supervision of the state. Subsequently, other states followed the Prussian example.

At the beginning of the twentieth century, a large number of small hospitals were founded at the initiative of public and private welfare organizations. Until the Second World War, hospital construction in Germany was left primarily to the market forces, which in most cases depended on local initiative. During the Second World War, however, things began to change. Because of the pressing need for medical care, the government forced existing hospitals to develop ambulatory care facilities, which, it should be mentioned, had not been a part of the average German hospital until then (except for some university teaching hospitals, which had had outpatient care facilities for a long time). The war also brought about other changes. Some 80 percent of the hospitals had been destroyed by the end of the war. There was a pressing need to reconstruct the destroyed hospitals and to use those still available—mainly small hospitals—in the most efficient way. The lack of available facilities, combined with the large number of physicians either returning from the war or emerging from medical school, where they had gone in great numbers to avoid the draft, made it absolutely essential to open up all available facilities to any practicing physician. Hospital specialists began to press for bed renewal, either through reconstruction or through the updating of intact facilities to reflect medical developments, an updating which had been delayed because of the war. This pressure from the physicians was increased by the absence of ambulatory care facilities. Such facilities had traditionally been uncommon in hospitals because of the reimbursement policies of sickness funds. Thus, hospital staff and patients tended to use inpatient facilities for problems that could have been treated on an ambulatory basis. As early as the fifties, therefore, local governments, backed by physicians, started pressing not only for hospital renewal but also for larger and more specialized hospitals.

These reconstruction efforts, launched primarily through local initiative, were regulated only by the federal price regulations of August 31, 1954. Inadvertently, the regulated hospital per diem rates were far from covering costs, so that by the 1970s yearly hospital deficits were running as high as 2 billion Deutsche marks ($800 million). These post-World War II developments, combined with the lack of active federal intervention, resulted in: (1) a high bed/population ratio; (2) a widely varying and uncoordinated supply of hospital beds throughout the different states and regions; and (3) nearly catastrophic finances for the hospitals, aggravated by the federal price regulations of 1954.

The German Hospital Association was reinstated in 1949 as the association unifying nearly all federal and state hospital associations, and it developed into the main lobbying force concerned with general hospital policy in Germany. In 1953, at the initiative of this association and with the involvement of the Association of Department Heads, the Nurses Association of Germany, and the Association of German Hospital Administrators, the German Hospital Institute was founded to solve the hospitals' problems. From the start, the institute, whose role was primarily one of directing market forces, was active in stimulating better hospital planning, hospital construction programming, and improved physical layout. However, its effect has been more to disseminate information than to introduce a long-lasting solution.

The state governments and the federal government have also occasionally tried to bring about improvements. Different university departments, under state authority, have tried to improve hospital construction, and the federal government has supported special, mission-oriented research projects to improve hospital construction and hospital facilities. Despite these efforts, it was not until the Hospital Finance Act of 1972 that the federal government became actively involved in the physical development of better health care facilities.

The 1972 act dealt primarily with hospital financing and hospital planning. Essentially, hospitals were to receive financial aid on the condition that, with the help of their state governments, they provide some planning, programming, coordination, and cooperation. Hospitals that bypass the state-prepared hospital plans forgo these grants-in-aid. The subsidy mechanism is thus used as an incentive to planning.

Hospital planning under the 1972 act proceeds as follows. The states are responsible for need-oriented hospital inventories, for multi-year building plans based on these inventories, and for yearly detailed hospital building programs. These programs have to take into account the federal budget earmarked for hospital construction. Before October 1 of each year, the states must elaborate a hospital building program for the coming calendar year. The financial means required for the acquisition of medium- and short-term equipment have to be indicated. At the federal level, a Committee for Questions Concerning the Economic Security of the Hospitals (created by the Federal Minister of Youth, Family, and Health) advises on the technical aspects and coordination of the programs. The committee gives advice on the allocation of federal aid to remedy the maldistribution of hospital beds throughout the different states, and it is responsible for defining the general principles of an efficient hospital system, with services distributed according to the needs of the population. It can advise on all problems related to hospital tariffs and on the implementation of the 1972 act, in particular the coordination between federal and state objectives. While developing the hospital need inventories and the programs for hospital construction, the states must review the positions of all interest groups, such as the German Hospital Association, the high commissions of the sickness funds (employers and employees), and so on. Also, general federal planning criteria must be met. Unfortunately, because of deficiencies in information and background data, these criteria are still very limited. Some federal guidelines have been formulated on personnel utilization and average length of stay, but they date from 1969 and certainly do not have the power of law.

Furthermore, strong opposition has been raised to federal attempts to do away with local and specialized hospitals—that is, hospitals with fewer than a hundred beds—and to exclude special accommodations for private patients in the hospitals. Both the German Hospital Association and the Association of German Hospital Physicians fear that such attempts will only result in all first-rate specialists transferring to private and profit-making hospitals, thus creating a two-class delivery system. These organizations, backed up occasionally by other pressure groups such as local level political parties, have succeeded in preventing federal attempts to formulate guidelines or to intervene actively in resources development. Their main argument has been that government should not intervene in health service organization.

At present, all states have laws concerning hospital planning (Bundesministerium 1975, 7:4530). However, the level of detail and sophistication varies from state to state. Most state laws are still very much oriented towards basic resources—the number of beds to be constructed and the financial consequences. Some state laws go further, indicating the different hospital functions to be performed, including the type and size of the clinical functions. A few states have formulated policy guidelines on the integration of hospital facilities and non-hospital-based health care facilities. The investment flowing into hospital construction still receives the most attention in the laws of all states except Bavaria. Next in order of emphasis are the councils, technical advisory committees, and controlling agencies, which are considered necessary to supervise the process and to guarantee a democratic approach (these are included in seven states). The hospital program itself, which may or may not be binding, which may or may not specify hospitals, and which may or may not be elaborated by speciality and type of service, is regulated in six states. Four states have gone one step further and have touched on the management of hospital resources: hospital cooperation, admission policy, information systems, hospital management in structure and content, special privileges, and emergency services.

In general, no specific position has yet been reached concerning the regional distribution of hospitals. Recent research has revealed no differences in health status between states with a large number of beds per thousand and states with a rather small number of beds per thousand. Nevertheless, primarily for budgetary reasons, a national guideline on the number of beds per thousand is still being advocated. It is still unclear what this guideline should be. Everybody seems to agree that some balancing between "rich" and "poor" states is necessary, but the exact level remains undetermined.

Other Facilities

As a promising side effect of the 1972 act, state planning efforts have led to more widespread public discussion of the whole question of health care delivery. Health facility planning in general is being discussed, rather than the planning of specific facilities, health care reorganization rather than hospital development, and integrated health care delivery rather than hospital care. The need for new types of health care facilities has been recognized and is being openly discussed, not only within university and nonuniversity health services research centers, but also in the public media and in political forums. Extended-care facilities and health care or medical centers are the two types of facilities currently receiving most attention. However, discussions have not yet reached the pragmatic stage, and are still focused on health care models—including structure, organization, financing, and remuneration schemes. Some tentative models have been proposed by interested parties (hospital organizations, insurance companies, physician organizations). Some state experiments have also been planned (for example, in Berlin and Bremen), involving the German Hospital Association and the Trade Association Sickness Funds, although none have yet been started. Experiments are also planned in some cities (Köln-Chorweiler). The main stumbling block seems to be the physicians' fear of "socialized" medicine as it has evolved in Sweden and the United Kingdom, which they feel might result from an integration of ambulatory and hospital care.

The topic of group practices is also being discussed. Whether group practices should be homogeneous (involving one speciality) or heterogeneous (involving more specialities), is unclear; the facilities required by these two types are recognized to be quite different. Interestingly, the sickness funds affiliated physician groups have opposed the idea of heterogeneous group practices, since they fear that such practices will only aggravate competition among different medical specialities.

Information Resources

Health Research

Health research in Germany has a long tradition of excellent researchers producing excellent results. In 1911, the government made its first attempt to organize health research. The Emperor Wilhelm Society was founded as a specific health research institute outside the universities, to provide excellent laboratory facilities to a limited number of scientists. Eventually renamed the Max Planck Society, this nonprofit organization today comprises a large number of research institutes in Germany. Although originally funded by the national government and reorganized financially by the Königstein Agreement of 1948, the society has maintained its autonomy in management and policy formulation. The Königstein Agreement resulted in a tripartite breakdown of research institutes: first, those funded by the states on an individual basis; second, those funded by all states (Königstein Agreement institutes); and third, those funded partly by the states and partly by the federal government (Max Planck Society institutes) (Wissenschaftsrat 1965). Of the fifty-two Max Planck Society institutes in 1971, twenty-eight belonged to the section for biology and medicine, which includes about 35 percent of the 4,000 scientists now working in the society (Fleischhauer 1973, p. 89). The government's influence in the society is rather subtle: the senate, the society's highest executive body, always includes, in addition to scientists, eminent individuals from state and federal government and from industry and commerce.

Immediately after the Second World War, the German Research Society was founded as an independent association to coordinate the whole research sector by providing grants for particular projects. The German Research Society is financed equally by the federal and state governments, but it is also supported by industry and private sources. About one-third of its financial aid goes to biomedical research—in 1969, about 30 million Deutsche marks or $12 million (Bundesministerium 1972). The division of this society into specialized subcommittees to examine proposals and approve grants tends to confirm research patterns in traditional disciplines. Hence, the society was for a long time unable to influence university structures or to reorient research.

In 1952, the German Research Society launched a priority procedure to enable German science to fill the gaps resulting from the losses of the Second World War. The society itself selects priority research sectors that it believes merit exceptional assistance, and it decides for itself if projected goals have been attained. The development of molecular biology and the institution of a national network of computer centers owe their success to this procedure. Nevertheless, neither the normal grant procedure nor the priority procedure has been successful in reorienting research in general, or biomedical research in particular. Nor has the German Research Society brought about a coordination among university research, industry research, and other research activities. Because of this impasse, in 1957 the president of the Federal Republic of Germany created a new advisory body: the Science Council. Since its inception, the Science Council has advocated the creation and development of concentrated research centers in the German universities. As a result, a special-research-sectors program was initiated in 1968, which added to the Science Council's consultative function an increasingly important executive responsibility for research, including medical research. Proposals for special research sectors may come through various channels. This multi-channel approach reflects the need to reconcile the interests of the federal government, the states, the universities, and any party concerned. Money is allocated from a special fund, provided two-thirds by the Federal government and one-third by the state government. Some twenty-six of the seventy special research sectors funded in 1970 were in biomedical research.

The Federal Health Bureau is an institution that works for the government in such fields as drugs (where it is comparable to the United States Food and Drug Administration), narcotics, and special areas of public health such as epidemiology, nuclear medicine, and toxicology. The Bureau also runs the Institute for Social Medicine and Epidemiology, founded in 1969, which keeps track of standard morbidity, mortality, and epidemiologic data in Germany. In accordance with the general belief that the bureau's role should be expanding, its budget has been increased in recent years to 210 million Deutsche marks per annum ($84 million).

While the 1948 Königstein Agreement redistributed influence over research policy to the state governments, as opposed to the federal government, in recent years the federal government's coordinating role has increased, basically because of increased financial leverage in research matters, and because the states themselves have been unable to develop a coordinated research policy.

Health Statistics

In the development of health information systems, the German government has emphasized health insurance information, and it has depended on the states for the collection of the information. Because of the dependence on state cooperation, the health information system is less coherent and less well developed than in neighboring countries, although certain recent attempts at dispersed and independent sites are technically promising. The 1931 agreement between the medical profession and the sickness funds did introduce a promising mechanism to monitor physician activity, but no national effort has been made to utilize this mechanism to improve health services. Four major funds cooperated in the sixties to permit a physician belonging to one of the funds automatically to belong to the other three, but no real exchange of data or merging of data banks took place. Hence, most health information is of a traditional nature, and relates not so much to health as to the characteristics and activities of health care providers, of which hospitals are, as in other countries, the best documented.

The number and type of physicians and hospitals are fairly well known and the figures are regularly updated by the Federal Bureau for Statistics. This bureau also handles traditional epidemiological statistics, such as statistics on mortality, tuberculosis, and communicable diseases, in cooperation with the Federal Health Bureau of the Ministry of Youth, Family, and Health. However, little is known about other morbidity characteristics or about patient use of the different elements of the health care system. To elicit this type of information, the ministry has organized several sample surveys:

Ten percent of the population was surveyed in April 1966 to determine illness and accident incidence rates by age, sex, and other factors. This sample was prepared, drawn up, and investigated within the framework of the federal government's census statistics.

Hospital morbidity was surveyed in three Hessen hospitals in 1964.

A further attempt was made to improve morbidity and mortality statistics in 1967 and 1968, in a study of four hospitals affiliated
with the Goethe University in Frankfurt.
A special survey was made of cardiac infarct incidence rates from
1958 to 1968 in Hamburg.

The federal ministry has stressed the need for a more detailed and
more flexible health information system, and several attempts have
already been made to bring this about. In a policy statement in October 1969, Chancellor Willy Brandt identified social medicine as an
area of priority. The Federal Institute for Social Medicine and Epidemiology, subsequently established, was given the specific task of
developing the information systems necessary for epidemiological
research and preventive medicine. Several organizations have been
founded with federal help to undertake the specific task of disseminating health related information:

—The German Institute for Medical Documentation and Information, concerned with the progress and results of biomedical research.
—The Institute for Documentation and Information on Social Medicine and Public Health, affiliated with the German Research Society, is sponsored by the Minister for Health, Labor, and Social
Affairs of Nord-Rhein-Westphalen and was founded in 1966;
this institute concentrates on social medicine and public health
research findings and progress.
—The German Hospital Institute Documentation Center provides
financial aid to explore and develop a hospitals-related information system.

In addition, the most recent policy statements published by the Federal Ministry of Youth, Family, and Health list the development of
census data relevant to health care planning, including health care
personnel planning, as one of five top priorities.

Cost data are primarily in the hands of the sickness funds. The
original Hospital Finance Bill submitted by the federal minister of
youth, family, and health on August 4, 1970, contained several ref-
erences to the development of economically efficient hospitals and
the management instruments that should be developed to achieve
them; but the act passed on June 29, 1972, limited itself to stating
the goals and left out all reference to specific instruments. This ab-

sence is said to have been brought about by the German Hospital Association (DKG) and the Hospital Physician Association. At any rate, the German Hospital Institute, in association with the Hospital Association, is still developing instruments for interhospital cost comparison and cost information. Health cost data are rather "soft" in Germany, hence links between illness incidence and cost data, or cost-benefit analysis, have not so far been established.

In Retrospect

Germany was the first country to embark on the daring social experiment of introducing national health insurance. In doing so it inspired other countries such as Great Britain and Japan. It was the only country in the world that ever enacted national health insurance without noticeable opposition from the medical profession. But that opposition ultimately arose, bringing with it the issues and principles that the medical profession would from then on use in its confrontations with governments throughout the world over the question of health insurance. Germany thus became the archetype of a compulsory contributory health insurance system, one lowering financial barriers in the access to care by a largely independent provider community rewarded by fee-for-service. The archetype is now being challenged by the government, which is using regulatory pressure in an effort to improve the supply and distribution of health resources and to control the expanding costs of health care.

3 | England and Wales

For England and Wales, which were chosen as representative of Great Britain, the important episodes in the development of national health insurance were self-evident. A limited health insurance scheme, following the Bismarckian model, was introduced in 1911 as part of a liberal reform program inspired by David Lloyd George and Winston Churchill (National Insurance Act 1911). In 1946 it was decided not to extend the scheme to the entire population, as the French had decided to do about that time, but to abolish it. Some ignorant of British history and life have interpreted this decision as revolutionary (Eckstein 1958, p. 2). This, however, is incorrect: a variety of circumstances—World War II, the position of specialists (consultants), the deplorable situation of the hospitals—combined, once again, with the diplomacy and energy of a brilliant politician, Aneurin Bevan, to pave the way for the creation of the National Health Service (National Health Service Act 1946). For more than twenty years, the NHS did not undergo fundamental changes, although proposals for reorganization were made from the early sixties on. On July 5, 1973, an act of Parliament drastically reorganized the NHS for the first time since its beginning in 1948 (NHS Reorganization Act 1973).

The 1911 National Health Insurance

The Advent of the Liberals

In the nineteenth century, individualist doctrines and self-help ideology (the Friendly Societies) played an important role in the provi-

sion of health care in the United Kingdom. Once the British realized, however, that private charity and self-help were ultimately
inadequate to meet the pressures placed upon them, a new concept
of society began to take shape. At the beginning of the twentieth
century the Liberal party managed to present a compromise between the individualist self-help doctrines and the socialistic alternative. This compromise was based on the traditional liberal respect
for the freedom of the individual, on the one hand, and on a limited
degree of collective control to protect those who had been shown unable to protect themselves, on the other. The ideal means for achieving this compromise was, in the eyes of the Liberal party, through
insurance. Insurance is essentially a personal matter, but it has to be
encouraged, enforced, and extended by the state to ensure its ade-
quacy (Bruce 1974, p. 172).

Sooner than expected, the Liberal party had the opportunity to
enact its program: the election of 1906 resulted in a stupendous Liberal victory and a sizable majority in the House of Commons (Fraser
1973, p. 135). Asquith became prime minister in 1908, Lloyd George
became chancellor of the Exchequer, and Churchill became president of the Board of Trade. Both Lloyd George and Churchill carried Asquith's government forward into a progressive and active
social policy. The Old Age Pensions Act, 1908, the People's Budget
of 1909, and the National Insurance Act of 1911 can be considered
liberal reforms (Bruce 1974, p. 174). In 1905, the conservative government of Balfour had appointed the Royal Commission on the
Poor Laws and the Relief of Distress to investigate the working of
the Poor Laws. In its report in 1909, this commission showed a remarkable degree of unanimity in proposing a considerable reshap-
ing of the Poor Laws (Bruce 1974, p. 173). However, one of the
problems that divided the commission was medical care for the poor.
The central question was whether local medical care for indigents
should be merged with the functions of sanitary authorities into one
national medical service. Most members of the commission
vigorously opposed this idea, because it would lead to the state providing for practically everyone, to the detriment of voluntary organizations and private medical practice. It was also considered too
costly (Brand 1965, p. 196). A minority, however, especially Beatrice
Webb, favored a unified public health service, but with patients as-
signed to salaried general practitioners. In Mrs. Webb's opinion, a
salaried physician would not give in so rapidly to unreasonable de-

mands of patients. The establishment of a unified medical service would not, according to the minority report, involve a free provision of medical services to all applicants: charges could be levied to cover the cost of medical treatment for those who could afford it. The minority report had been drafted by both Beatrice and her husband Sidney Webb, although only Mrs. Webb was a member of the Poor Laws Commission. The Webbs, who always worked as a team, were members of the Fabian Society, which believed that state socialism would evolve gradually as government was confronted more and more by practical difficulties (Anderson 1972, p. 55).

The ideas behind the national health insurance scheme of 1911 were deeply influenced by the Poor Laws reports of 1909. The introduction of the scheme actually followed the recommendation by the Royal Commission on the Poor Laws that medical assitance should be organized on a provident basis (Levy 1944, p. 3). Another important liberal reform that paved the way for the National Insurance Act was the so-called People's Budget of 1909. One of its purposes was to raise money for social needs through special taxes on higher incomes and through graduated income taxes (Bruce 1974, p. 210). Lloyd George was drawn towards the insurance principle by his desire to extend to widows and orphans the state pension for elderly people, which had previously been paid entirely out of general revenue. But such an extension would have been so costly that it could never be financed by taxation alone. So he turned to insurance as a way to raise money. The Friendly Societies and the industrial assurance companies, which were active in the field, opposed his plans in order to protect their trade and their prerogative to pay, on death of the breadwinner, a lump sum or a widow's or orphan's pension. So Lloyd George dropped the idea of pensions financed by insurance and shifted his concern to sickness insurance.

Lloyd George favored the insurance principle not only because it was a simple method of gathering necessary revenue. Insurance also had a positive political appeal to him, and he used it as a political weapon (Fraser 1973, p. 152) to win votes at the expense of the Labor party. In doing so he imitated Bismarck. He had visited Germany in 1908 and he was "tremendously" impressed by what he had seen there. The British insurance scheme of 1911 was thus deeply influenced by the German example of national sickness insurance (Levy 1944, p. 3).

The principle of insurance was already accepted in Britain, having been established through the Friendly Societies, trade unions, medical aid societies, provident dispensaries, industrial assurance companies, and others. But in Lloyd George's point of view, these initiatives did not go far enough. Although more than six million people were covered by the Friendly Societies, and still more contributed to the collecting societies and industrial assurance companies, for a great part of the population insurance only provided a decent burial. Lloyd George was conscious of the problems of the worker who could not afford the services of a general practitioner and the medicines prescribed. Theoretically, he could have followed the Webbs' advice and attempted to introduce a national health service. But he knew that this would have provoked the Friendly Societies and the industrial assurance companies. His insight led him to placate these powerful forces by incorporating them as intermediaries in a national insurance scheme. He further saw the introduction of compulsory insurance as a way to remove a substantial section of the population from the Poor Law system without heavy expenditures from the Exchequer (Abel-Smith 1964, p. 237).

Coping with Opposition

Special interest groups definitely influenced the shape of the National Insurance Act (Levy 1944, p. 2). The Friendly Societies, insofar as they provided insurance for sickness, were afraid that they would suffer if a centralized state-administered scheme were introduced. Further, they wished to profit from an extension of their activities; if sickness insurance became compulsory, they would serve many more millions of people. The industrial assurance companies were startled by the prospect that Lloyd George might combine burial benefit with sickness benefit, as in the German scheme. Two outstanding concessions had to be made to bring these interests into the national health scheme and to secure their support for the whole measure. First, the activities of the existing voluntary associations and institutions were incorporated into the scheme by means of the so-called approved societies; second, burial benefits were excluded from the provision for sickness insurance (Levy 1944, p. 6).

The medical profession objected to the financial and administrative arrangements proposed and they wondered how their intellectual and financial independence could be maintained under the insurance scheme (Hogarth 1963, p. 16). Six "cardinal points" were defined and submitted to Lloyd George:

1. medical benefits for insured persons with an income under £ 2 a week only
2. free choice of doctor
3. medical benefits administered by insurance committees instead of the approved societies
4. exact method of payment decided by the doctors in each area
5. adequate remuneration
6. adequate professional representation in the operation of the schemes, at both local and central levels (Levy 1944, p. 6).

When the bill was finally accepted in the House of Commons, four of these six cardinal points were written into it. However, the doctors did not secure any change in the originally proposed income limit, and the vital question of amount of remuneration also remained unsolved. The government had offered six shillings per head per year, including drugs; the British Medical Association asked for eight shillings sixpence, excluding drugs. An inquiry into the actual income of general practitioners was then carried out by William Plender, on behalf of the BMA and the government (Hogarth 1963, p. 17). He found that four shillings fivepence, including drugs, was the average annual income per physician per patient. The government offered seven shillings sixpence, later nine shillings, including drugs, but the BMA rejected the proposal. For many doctors, however, the fee of nine shillings per head signified a substantial raise in income, and increasing numbers of doctors began to accept work under the act, BMA opposition notwithstanding. In January 1913, national health insurance was under way. Levy remarks that "doctors resented in particular the fact that the proposal contained in the original bill for the establishment of a Local Health Committee in each county and county borough had been dropped. Each Committee was expected to consider 'the needs of the county and county borough with regard to all questions of public health, and may make such reports and recommendations with regard thereto as it may think fit'. But the local health committees were replaced by the insurance committees . . . [which] were not medical committees but insurance committees" (Levy 1944, p. 21).

The 1911 act did not directly affect the position of the hospitals, apart from a section permitting the approved societies to make grants to the voluntary hospitals. However, as soon as the bill was published, fears were expressed that the scheme would have serious indirect consequences for the hospitals. At a meeting of the British Hospital Association, in June 1911, it was pointed out that hospitals not only would lose subscriptions as a result of the bill, but also would have to pay contributions for their own employees. Rather rapidly, however, this concern about the effects of the act on hospital finances proved to be unfounded: the public continued to subscribe (Abel-Smith 1964, p. 239).

Provisions of the 1911 Act

National Health Insurance covered two distinct categories of insured persons:

1. compulsory contributors: all persons between the ages of sixteen and sixty-five gainfully occupied in certain classes of employment remunerated at no more than £ 160 per year.
2. voluntary contributors: all persons of age sixteen and upwards who did not belong to either of the compulsory contributor classes, but who were engaged in some other regular occupation, or had been compulsory contributors for at least five years.

Insurance was financed seven-ninths (in case of women, three-quarters) by the contributors and two-ninths (women, one-quarter) by Parliament. The contributions payable by the employer were sevenpence a week for men, sixpence a week for women. Threepence a week were to be paid by the employer, fourpence a week by a male contributor, and threepence a week by a female. The employer actually paid both amounts but was entitled to recover the amount of the employee's contribution by deduction from his wage. The contribution of voluntary contributors was at a rate appropriate to their age at the date of entry into insurance.

The benefits offered were medical benefits (medical treatment and attendance, proper and sufficient medicines, medical and surgical appliances as prescribed), sanatorium benefits (treatment when suffering from tuberculosis, including stay in sanatorium), sickness benefits; disability benefits, and maternity benefits. For medical benefits, a waiting period of six months after entry into the scheme was mandatory. Medical and sanatorium benefits were in all cases administered by and through the insurance committees in every county or county borough. Three-fifths of the committee membership were insured persons, and each committee included two physicians; all members had to be residents of the county or county borough. The insurance committee was obliged to consult the local medical committee, once it was recognized as representing the medical practitioners living in the county or county borough, on all questions affecting the administration of medical benefits. All the contributions and all the money from Parliament was paid into the National Health Insurance Fund.

A Case of Income Insurance?

Lloyd George's intentions in introducing the insurance scheme have been interpreted in many different ways. Thus, Honingsbaum writes: "Professor Bentley Gilbert . . . was completely wrong when it came to interpretation. Lloyd George, he claimed, wanted 'to replace lost income, not to cure sickness' but Sir George Newman (who was in a position to know) has suggested otherwise. The Chancellor, Newman once wrote, 'appeared to be handling a finance measure— as indeed he was—but it was still more a health measure, and he knew it'" (Honingsbaum 1970, p. 12). On this subject Levy states: "It was only natural that he (Lloyd George) . . . laid emphasis upon the improvement in health to be expected from N.H.I. It was an argument which nobody could resist in good faith." He continues that those who criticized the act for not carrying with it a comprehensive, uniform scheme for health improvement, entirely overlooked that the object of the act was in the first place "to provide insurance against loss of health" and only in the second place "for the prevention and cure of sickness" (Levy 1944, p. 21).

The act itself contained some measures for the development of health resources. A very important innovation was included in Section 16. Subsection 2 of this section stated that, out of the money contributed by Parliament for each insured person, one penny should be contributed annually to the expenses of sanatorium benefits; and it continued that the insurance commissioners could retain the whole or any part of that contribution "for the purposes of research." In this rather indirect way, a national fund for medical research was created, which ultimately resulted in the important Medical Research Council. Section 21 of the 1911 act provided that:

"It shall be lawful . . . for an insurance committee to grant such subscriptions or donations as it may think fit to hospitals, dispensaries and other charitable institutions, or for the support of district nurses and to appoint nurses for the purpose of visiting and nursing insured persons." However, according to Abel-Smith, Section 21 had negligible effects on health resources development.

Section 60 required the insurance committees to make reports on the health of insured persons and to furnish statistical and other returns; further, they could organize lectures and publish information on questions relating to health. Section 64.4 further prescribed that: "An insurance committee may, with the consent of the insurance commissioners, enter into agreements with any person or authority that, in consideration of such persons or such authority providing treatment in a sanatorium, the committee will contribute out of the funds available for sanatorium benefits towards the maintenance of the institution . . . such annual or other payments . . . as may be agreed."

Towards a National Health Service

The Prewar Problems

By 1939, about 50 percent of the population were paying for general practitioner services through the National Insurance scheme, which had undergone no serious structural changes since 1911. In 1929, the British Medical Association, in its "Proposal for a General Medical Service for the Nation," had argued that the scheme should be extended to dependents of insured persons and to persons using the Poor Law domiciliary services; further, the services provided should be extended to include maternity and specialist services. Extension of benefits and coverage had been proposed even earlier, by the Royal Commission on the National Health Insurance in 1926 and in the revised 1929 BMA proposal in 1938. Nevertheless, in 1939 the scheme continued to provide more or less the same benefits as in 1911: "The additions that have been made here and there in the case of certain services and some rich societies, still leave a wide vacuum in the most important fields: e.g. nursing, treatment of tuberculosis, appliances or artificial limbs, maternity benefits, treatment by specialist, hospital treatment" (Levy 1944, p. 332).

From the patients' point of view, a comprehensive service existed only for those who could pay, with the result that many had to go without medical care or without the appropriate medical care. General practitioners claimed to be overworked, isolated from one another and from hospitals, and badly distributed geographically (Willcocks 1967, p. 21). In 1939 hospital services were provided either by local authorities or by voluntary bodies, the local authority hospitals containing some 143,000 beds, and the more numerous voluntary hospitals about 72,000 beds. The local authorities provided mainly fever, isolation, and mental hospitals, although after the Local Government Act of 1929—which merged the Poor Law authorities and the local authorities by handing over the powers, duties, and institutions of the former to the latter—local authorities expanded their work with general hospitals.

The local authorities had a statutory duty to admit all sick persons requiring hospital treatment, while the voluntary hospitals, whose patients either paid (in person or through some insurance system) or were treated free, could pick and choose their patients (Abel-Smith 1964, p. 430). The many hospital authorities seldom cooperated to achieve a rational provision of services in any area. The 1937 Report of the Voluntary Hospitals Commission (the Sankey Report) and the 1938 British Medical Association document "A General Medical Service for the Nation" both proposed regional coordinating machinery for the provision of hospital services; but such proposals were never implemented. The BMA refrained from recommending that hospital treatment be included in the benefit package, mainly because it thought it unfeasible to attempt to guarantee sufficient accommodation (Abel-Smith 1964, p. 348). In 1939, the most serious deficiencies in hospital services were (Willcocks 1967, p. 22) inadequate accommodation, shortage and maldistribution of specialists, and lack of coordination among hospitals; the voluntary hospitals also had growing financial difficulties.

The Influence of World War II

R. Titmuss discusses at length the influence of modern warfare on social policy in general and on the provision of health care in particular. He identifies a dominating development in modern war: a state's increasing concern with the biological characteristics of its people (Titmuss 1958, ch. 4). According to him, this concern had developed in different stages. At first, the state was interested in the number of men available for battle, which led to a national census and interest in vital statistics. Then, qualitative standards were adopted and applied to recruits. Finally, public concern about the fitness of recruits widened to include the health and well-being of the whole population and, in particular, of children (the next generation of recruits). Titmuss believes that the Boer War stimulated the personal health movement that eventually led to the National Health Service in 1948. During the First World War, a first free national health service was introduced, when facilities were offered to civilians and soldiers alike for the treatment and prevention of venereal diseases. Still another stage in this development was reached during World War II, since the war required the total participation of all citizens. Not only was it necessary for the state to safeguard the people's physical health for reasons of defense, but mobilizing the entire population required that "we had something better to offer than had our enemies—not only during but also after the war." Mass mobilization in fact required an increase of social discipline; this discipline was tolerable if, and only if, social inequalities were reduced to a tolerable level. Mass mobilization called for social justice, for the abolition of privileges, for a more equitable distribution of income and wealth, and for drastic changes in the economic and social life of the country. These considerations led Titmuss to state that "The N.H.S. Act in 1946 was, in part, an expression of this wartime mood for justice and equality of opportunity" (Titmuss, p. 317). The Emergency Medical Service created in 1938 had an important influence on the provision of health care in the United Kingdom. Originally the EMS was intended to cope with air raid casualties and to care for service men and evacuated children. But its scope was widened during the war. First, it was made responsible for hospital patients who were moved into the country to make room for casualties in the city. In September 1940, the Ministry of Health decided to make beds available "to aged and infirm persons found in public shelters and rest centers." Then, between 1940 and 1942, the scope of the EMS was widened again, to include more civilians: munition workers, at the end of 1940, and all evacuated and homeless people, in 1941. And in July 1942, the ministry decided to allow more civilian patients to be "transferred" to the EMS from hospitals with waiting lists (Abel-Smith 1964, p. 431).

The EMS used both voluntary and local-authority institutions. Voluntary hospitals were paid for their services and received subsidies for keeping their beds empty for casualties. (This sometimes had very odd consequences. Since any reduction in casualty beds meant a reduction in subsidy, voluntary hospitals tended to keep beds empty rather than to admit civilian cases; as a result, local authority hospitals became overcrowded.) During the war, the voluntary hospitals increased their reserves by £ 10 million. All hospitals became heavily dependent on the central government to pay for their maintenance expenditures; it was realized that if the higher standard of service that had been reached during the war was to be maintained in peacetime, much higher expenditures would be needed. On the other hand, as Abel-Smith states, "expenditures on medical care came to be regarded less as a form of consumption and more as a positive investment in the war effort" (Abel-Smith 1964, p. 437). When plans for the EMS were made in 1938, it was estimated that one to three million hospital beds would be necessary for air raid casualties alone. Faced with this enormous prospective demand, the Ministry of Health decided to carry out the first official survey of the conditions of hospitals in Britain. The results of this survey were disturbing (Abel-Smith 1964, p. 425). Some of the investigators— among them outstanding clinicians—were shocked by the existing situation in the hospitals and became the first protagonists of a National Hospital Service as part of the NHS.

Another consequence of the EMS was the redistribution of specialists from well-provided metropolitan and teaching hospitals into ordinary local hospitals, which were often small and very poorly equipped. The specialists expressed their horrified reactions in many letters to the medical press. No doubt this was one of the factors behind the decision of Ernest Brown, the minister of health of the wartime coalition government in 1941, to set up a comprehensive hospital service after the war, which would be available for all, making use of both voluntary and local government hospitals (Willcocks 1967, p. 22). The Beveridge Report broadened the idea of a hospital service into a health service. The principal politician pushing for Beveridge to prepare his now famous report was Clement Attlee, head of the Labor party during World War II. Attlee had been acutely aware of the civil unrest provoked by returning soldiers after World War I; he believed that the general strike of 1921 reflected much of their discontent and disillusionment with civilian life. He was determined that the British system of education and health should be more responsive to the needs of the veterans and their families. The Beveridge Committee (a small interdepartmental committee) was set up "to undertake a survey of the existing national scheme of social insurance and allied services." Health services were not explicitly within Beveridge's ambit, but his proposals for an extension and coordination of the social insurance schemes were based upon the assumption that there would be a comprehensive national health service.

The Beveridge Report was debated in Parliament in February 1943. The government accepted the idea of a reorganized and comprehensive health service that would serve all the people, and which would include hospital treatment. In October 1941 the government had advanced the idea of a comprehensive hospital service available to all who needed it, and by 1943 it was committed to preparing plans for a comprehensive health service that would cover the whole population (Abel-Smith 1964, p. 454). This commitment was enacted in 1946 in the National Health Service Act.

The Profession Divided

During World War II the British Medical Association continued to favor the "90 percent proposal"—the extension of health insurance coverage to dependents—that it had lobbied for from the early twenties. For the administration of this scheme, the BMA favored a public corporation, divorced from day-to-day political control and largely under the authority of fellow professionals, rather than a government department subject to supervision by Parliament. Seeing the future hospital service to be regionally controlled and planned, the BMA stressed that "regionalism must not be a regional system of local government." Cooperation among voluntary and local-authority hospitals was considered essential to prevent their nationalization. For the remuneration of the general practitioners, the BMA favored per capita payments (Willcocks 1967, p. 33).

By and large, the medical profession was divided in its stand vis-à-vis the NHS bill. The Royal Colleges, representing the interests of consultants, supported the bill's main provisions. The BMA, however, representing general practitioner interests, mounted a campaign to resist the bill. This campaign was outmaneuvered by Aneurin Bevan (Foot 1973).

Main Characteristics of the NHS Act

The 1946 NHS Act established a comprehensive health service designed to secure improvement in the physical and mental health "of the population of England and Wales." The benefits offered were: (1) hospital and specialist services, (2) health services related to social services provided by local authorities, and (3) other health services provided through executive councils (general medical and general dental services, pharmaceutical services, supplementary ophtalmic services). All the benefits were provided free of charge, except when the act expressly provided for the making and recovery of charges (for example, for accommodation in single rooms or small wards).

The central administrative responsibility "to provide the establishment of a comprehensive health service" was allocated to the minister of health. He was advised by a Central Health Services Council, representing the main groups in the service, and by specialized standing advisory committees. Apart from this general responsibility, the minister was also responsible for the provision of hospital and specialist services. To enable him to fulfill this task, almost all of the voluntary hospitals and all hospitals vested in local authorities were transferred to his authority. Voluntary hospitals designated as teaching hospitals were transferred to boards of governors.

On July 5, 1948, ownership of 2,688 out of 3,044 voluntary and municipal hospitals in England and Wales was thus vested in the minister of health. Only about 270 hospitals, mainly those belonging to Roman Catholic orders and a few others that could not conveniently be fitted into the national scheme, were allowed to remain in private hands; however, they too took part in the NHS by treating NHS patients under contractual arrangements (Ministry of Health, *National Health Services Notes,* 1:4; 12:1). Further, the minister had the power to constitute a Medical Practices Committee to ensure that the number of general practitioners in the areas of the executive councils was adequate. Any doctor who wished to take up an NHS practice had first to receive the consent of the Medical Practices Committee.

The Minister and his officials obviously could not manage or plan the service in detail from London; they required the assistance of regional or local bodies. To make the health service acceptable to the medical profession, medical syndicalism was built into these bodies, and the local authorities and the hospitals were also given a share of the power. Thus, the service had a tripartite structure: the hospital and specialist services, local-authority health services, and general medical services.

For the hospital and specialist services, England was divided into fourteen large hospital regions, while Wales itself became one hospital region. Regional Hospital Boards (RHB's) were established. The RHB's were responsible—under the general guidance of the minister—for planning and coordinating the development of hospital and specialist services for their region and for supervising their administration, particularly their expenditures. Further, they had to appoint Hospital Management Committees (HMC's). The HMC's in fact undertook the day-to-day running of the hospitals, under the general guidance of the RHB's. In general, each HMC administered a group of hospitals (*National Health Services Notes,* 12:3). Separate arrangements were introduced for the administration of teaching hospitals. The board of governors of such a hospital was responsible for the combined functions of an RHB and an HMC.

The local health authorities had many functions. They had to provide and to maintain health centers, to staff them, and to provide a range of supporting services auxiliary to ordinary institutional and noninstitutional medical practice. The local authorities were the county councils and the county borough councils. Their NHS functions were part of their overall local function. However, for the purpose of the NHS Act, they acted through a health committee. At least a majority of the members of this committee also had to be members of the local authority.

In the area of each health authority, an executive council was constituted for the purpose of exercising functions with respect to general medical and dental services and pharmaceutical and ophthalmologic services. Closely related to the executive councils were the local medical, pharmaceutical, and dental committees (committees representing their respective professions). The executive council had to consult these committees on such occasions and to such extent as was prescribed. The most important duty of an executive council was to make arrangements with medical practitioners to be paid on a per capita basis for the provision of personal medical services. A dental estimates board was set up to approve estimates for the more expensive treatments submitted by dentists and to authorize payment for approved treatments. Most of the costs of the NHS were met from general revenue. Other, though limited, sources of finance were the weekly NHS contributions (introduced only in 1957) paid by all employees who had to pay National Insurance contributions, local taxation, which paid for about half the cost of the local authorities' health services, and partial charges to patients.

A Mandate for Resource Development

The 1946 act was the turning point for a country moving from a mixture of private services and gap-filling public services to a system that set out to meet all needs insofar as they could be met. Naturally, the way in which these services were put together in 1948 depended upon what existed before (Godber 1975, p. 3). While the NHS act extended and developed the system of general practitioner services that had evolved under national health insurance, for the hospital and specialist services a whole new system of planning and administration was created in an attempt to rationalize the inherited system.

The 1946 act itself did not include many specific measures for health resources development, which is typical of the British approach to legislation. Article 1 of the NHS act charged the minister of health with "the duty . . . to provide the establishment in England and Wales of a comprehensive health service . . . and for that purpose to provide or secure the effective provision of services in accordance with the provision of this Act." Thus, the act contained a continuous and overall mandate for health resources development, but only in the form of a general framework to be filled by statutory regulations, which are easier to adapt to changing circumstances than an act of Parliament. Furthermore, circumstances made it impossible for the minister to fulfill his duty at once. The first decade after the war was one of considerable material shortage. With all the other capital reconstruction work required in the country, there was little to spare for hospitals. Funds, building materials, and labor for health purposes were minimal (Godber 1975, p. 25). Successive ministers, given their limited financial allocations, continued to postpone all but the most essential capital development. Money could not be found to build hospitals until the sixties.

Apart from the broad mandate stated in Article 1, the 1946 act did contain a few specific measures on health resources development—for instance, a mechanism for the spatial redistribution of general practitioners. But all such measures are fundamentally linked to one another through Article 1. As Sir George Godber wrote to the authors of this study: "This statute is so framed that the policies which are never spelled out in detail can be implemented without change in the law for many years. That explains the lack of health resources development in the act. It is not the place for it."

The National Health Service Reorganization Act, 1973

Obsolete Tripartition

In 1956, the Gillebaud Report (Ministry of Health 1956) revealed that many people were critical of the tripartite structure of the NHS and were concerned that the NHS might develop into a national hospital scheme, with overemphasis on curative medicine, instead of a real national health service in which prevention would play as important a role as cure (British Medical Association 1970, p. 25). However, the Gillebaud Report did not propose any fundamental change in the structure of the NHS. In 1962, the Medical Services Review Committee (a wholly professional committee under the chairmanship of Arthur Porritt) recommended that the responsibility for administration and coordination of all medical and allied services in any one area should be in the hands of a single area authority: the Area Health Board (Chester, p. 5). On November 6, 1967, the minister of health, Keith Robinson, announced that he had decided to make a careful examination of the administrative structure of the medical and related services for which he was responsible. His first official proposal regarding reorganization was published under a Labor government in 1968 as a "green paper" (referred to as Green Paper One) (Robinson 1968). In 1970, Robinson's successor, Richard Crossman, secretary of state for social services, published Green Paper Two (Crossman 1970). Then, the Conservative government in 1971 published a "consultative document," which led to the white paper of August 1972, published by Keith Joseph, secretary of state for social services (Joseph 1972), upon which the eventual NHS reorganization bill and NHS reorganization act were based. The central theme of both green papers was the same: the need to weld together, at every level, the three parts of the NHS—hospital and specialist services, local authority health services, and general medical services—to form an integrated service, instead of the multiplicity of authorities involved in the existing arrangements: Regional Hospital Boards, Hospital Management Committees, boards of governors, executive councils, local authorities, the ministry (Robinson 1968; Crossman 1970). In 1946, the tripartite, functional organization of the NHS had been considered reasonable and inevitable (Chester, p. 3). In the 1960s, however, this structure had emerged as "fundamentally unsound." Both the green papers give examples of confused and overlapping responsibility, uncoordinated services, absence of joint planning, and so on. The green papers proposed a single authority for each area, replacing the existing separate administrative bodies and taking over some important functions of the local health authorities. The two papers largely dealt with the problems of the relationships between the new area authorities and the local authorities, on the one hand (more particularly with the underlying question of whether health and social services should be provided by an integrated health service), and the relationship between the area authorities and the central government, on the other hand. According to Green Paper One, there should have been only one single planning agency: the central government (Robinson 1968, p. 12). Green Paper Two, however, proposed "regional health councils," whose most important function would have been planning. The area authorities were considered too small to function as planning units. Regarding the relationship between the area authority and the local authority, an important function was to be exercised by the "community physician." The two green papers considered him as a kind of bridge between these authorities, an adviser who could survey the general pattern of care in both the hospitals and the community (Crossman 1970, p. 14).

Scope and Content of the Reorganization

The main purposes of the 1973 Reorganization Act were:

1. To unify the local administration of the NHS under new health authorities responsible for the whole field of health care. The act requires the secretary of state to establish Regional Health Authorities and Area Health Authorities (RHA's and AHA's); the latter may vary in function according to whether they provide substantial facilities to support university medical and dental education. The AHA's are required to establish Family Practitioner Committees, while the secretary of state can establish Special Health Authorities for special purposes. The relation between

these administrative bodies is based upon the principle of delegation: the secretary of state, who has the general duty to provide for a comprehensive NHS, may direct an RHA or an AHA to exercise on his behalf specific functions relating to the NHS. An RHA can similarly direct AHA's. Family Practitioner Committees have the duty to administer, on behalf of the AHA's, the provision of general medical and dental services and general ophthalmic and pharmaceutical services.

2. To provide means in each area for representing the interests of the community. To this purpose, Community Health Councils were established. At least half of the membership of a council must consist of persons appointed by local authorities, at least one-third must be appointed by voluntary organizations, and one-sixth by the RHA of the area. The councils have to "represent the interest of the public in health services in their district."

3. To ensure that the views of the health professions are given full weight in the planning and the management of services. Therefore, the 1973 Reorganization Act, like the 1946 NHS Act, provides statutory recognition of local advisory committees representing the health care professions. Further, the health professions are represented in the newly established authorities.

4. To continue the NHS responsibility to provide facilities for the medical and teaching functions of universities. The secretary of state has the duty to make available those facilities reasonably required by any university that has a medical or dental school, in connection with clinical teaching and research and clinical dentistry.

5. To provide collaboration between the NHS and the social services provided by local authorities and between the NHS and voluntary organizations. Health authorities and local authorities have to cooperate to secure and advance the health and the social welfare of the people of England and Wales. Therefore, Joint Consultative Committees are to be established to advise the AHA's and the local authorities on the performance of their duties and on the planning and operation of services of common concern. More specifically, the secretary of state can make available to local authorities goods, materials, facilities, and services of persons employed by the secretary of state or by a health authority; on the other hand, local authorities can make available to health authorities the services of persons they employ. The secretary of state can

make arrangements with any person or body, including voluntary organizations, for that person or body to provide any service under the NHS Act.

6. To provide for the appointment of Health Service Commissioners for England and Wales to investigate complaints against health authorities. Although in the past the great majority of complaints were—according to the government—satifactorily dealt with by the existing health authorities, some critics said that the citizen should be able to refer to an entirely independent authority if he remained dissatisfied with the action taken by the health authority. This was considered as an important expansion of the ombudsman principle (Joseph 1972, app. II).

Position of the BMA

The BMA regretted the distinction between health and social services retained in the white paper, but was prepared to accept the general principle upon which the government had decided to define the administrative distinction. The BMA was also satisfied with the outline of the responsibilities of the community physicians. The BMA was divided on the question of whether an intermediate (RHA) level, between the minister and the area (AHA), should be established. In 1973, when the NHS reorganization bill became law, the BMA did not appear discontented with the results: there was no interference with clinical freedom by management or the new NHS ombudsman; there was a statutory advisory machinery, the composition of which would be determined largely by the medical profession; the independent contractor status of the general practitioner was preserved; and the School Health Service was transferred from the local authorities to the new health authorities (British Medical Association 1973, p. 29).

A New Departure for Resource Development

The integrated new managerial structure of the NHS was designed as a framework within which reorganization of NHS planning and budgeting could be implemented. Future resources development would depend fundamentally on the effectiveness of these revised planning and budgeting systems. Whereas the unified organizational structure was instituted on April 1, 1974, the new planning and budgeting system was delayed for two years and only was started on April 1, 1976, by the Department of Health and Social Security (DHSS). This new NHS planning and budgeting system replaced the compartmental ad hoc plans and budgets that had formerly been employed. It was based on a broader DHSS planning system, the skeleton of which was determined by three formal procedures.

1. The Public Expenditure Survey Systems (PESS) were introduced in 1961 and consist of multi-year public expenditure forecasts to be developed each year by government departments (English 1976, p. 166).
2. The Programme Budget system was introduced in the DHSS in 1970 and is defined as follows: "It is not a complex technique but a crude method of costing policies based on past expenditure. Its central purpose is to enable the Department to cost policies for service development across the board, so that priorities can be considered within realistic financial contraints. The Programme Budget is neither a forecast nor a plan: it is a way of exploring possible future strategies for development" (Department of Health and Social Security 1976). A very important characteristic of the Programme Budget is that it attempts to group expenditure around so-called "client groups," that is, the most important groups of users—the elderly and the physically and mentally handicapped—instead of around the different categories of health care providers and facilities.
3. The preparation of long-term policies within the DHSS was systematically coordinated, starting in 1973 (Van de Vijsel 1977).

Out of these three formal procedures a DHSS planning system has emerged, the first results of which appeared in 1976 through the publication of *Priorities for Health and Personal Social Services in England, A Consultative Document*. This document embodies a major new approach to planning (Department of Health and Social Security 1976, p. iii). However, the document is not merely the outcome of new planning ideas, but also suggests a new planning cycle for the NHS. For this reason, the document has been entitled "consultative"; the strategy it contains has to be validated by the NHS planning process that was introduced on April 1, 1976, after the publication of the document. That is why the *Consultative Document* is regarded as "a new departure" (Department of Health and Social Security 1976, p. 1). According to the document, the NHS planning system interacts with the DHSS planning system in that the DHSS system develops national guidelines for the Regional and Area health authorities and districts, where the NHS planning then takes place. These departmental guidelines have a twofold character, because they indicate the available financial resources and the targets and priorities in relation to development and utilization of health resources.

Human Resources

Health Manpower

The first government intervention into the development of health manpower concerned the training of physicians. The Medical Act of 1858 set up a General Council for Medical Education—later called the General Medical Council—with powers to supervise physicians' training. Although there was no provision to ensure that this council would represent the profession as a whole, its members were to be appointed partly by the medical associations. An identical trend of cooperation between the government and the professions took place in nursing and midwifery. The Midwives Act of 1902 set up a Central Midwives Board, consisting of four doctors and five other persons, one of whom was to be appointed by the Royal British Nurses Association. This board had to prescribe the conditions of training. The Nurses Registration Act of 1919 set up a General Nursing Council, which consisted of nine lay members and sixteen nurses. This council was empowered to develop training schemes. Thus, the government health manpower policy started with educational schemes for different health professions, the professional organizations of which pushed the government to take initiative, especially in the case of the nurses, whose professional organizations even drafted a bill.

From the time of its formation, the Ministry of Health has been continuously involved in this kind of health manpower policy and has even subsidized educational schemes. As Watkin points out, in 1919 the newly established Ministry of Health and the Board of Education jointly sponsored a two-year training course for health visitors for home care (Watkin 1975, p. 53). Whether the education of health care personnel should be the responsibility of the Department of Health or the Department of Education has always been a matter of discussion. When discussing the Briggs Report on Nursing, 1972, Watkin writes that "a number of bodies had urged the committee that nursing and midwifery education should be made the responsibility of the Department of Education and Science and that all nursing and midwifery students should be integrated into the higher education system." But the Briggs Report rejected these arguments and recommended "that in order for educational policies to be properly related to long-term manpower needs, overall responsibility should remain with the Health Department" (Watkin 1975, p. 328).

In addition to these professional and scientific organizations (such as the Royal Colleges) and the government, private persons and groups have also been involved in human resources development. Florence Nightingale set an example that led to the development of the nursing profession, and one of the first advisory committees on health professions was the Commission on Nursing set up in 1930 by the owners of *The Lancet* (Watkin 1975, p. 285). The 1911 National Health Insurance Act influenced the development of general practitioners to the extent that Titmuss has, in retrospect, called it "the general practitioner's act" (Titmuss, p. 300). By focusing solely on the services of general practitioners, it emphasized the division between general practitioners and consultants. The object of the act was to consolidate and strengthen the position of the general practitioner. It gave the average doctor a much better income, and it brought the greater mass of wage earners into contact with doctors. According to Rosemary Stevens, the act "established throughout society the concept of the family doctor" (Stevens 1966, p. 36). Titmuss does not share this opinion, however (Titmuss 1958, p. 173): "In the past (i.e. before 1948) 'family doctors' only existed for a small section of the population, mainly the inhabitants of relatively isolated rural areas and middle and upper middle class patients," and "many factors contributed, before 1948, to discouraging or preventing the G.P. from functioning as a family doctor."

This kind of health manpower policy, in which private initiative played a significant role, did not differ very much from the Continental pattern. But then, in 1946, the government took the vital decision that health services should be open to all on the basis of medical need. The ultimate difference between compulsory health insurance and a national health service depends on one characteristic: "In a public health service the government is explicitly responsible for the availability of sufficiently and adequately spread medical services, whereas this does not belong to the legal obligations of social insurance" (Van Langendonck 1975, p. 264). This decision made a real health manpower policy at least possible, if not necessary.

Physicians

The 1946 NHS Act contained a mechanism for the geographical redistribution of general practitioners. The Medical Practices Committee could refuse an application for practice in a given area if the number of doctors in that area was already considered to be sufficient, or an application could be approved for certain parts of an area only. When making a decision, the Medical Practices Committee had to take into account an applicant's desire to work in a group practice. A dissatisfied applicant had the right to appeal to the minister of health against the committee's decision. The executive councils had to make reports to the Medical Practices Committee on the number of general practitioners required, on the vacancies appearing in the list of general practitioners, and on the need to fill such vacancies. These reports enabled the committee to classify each area according to the number of doctors practicing there, on the basis, essentially, of statistical criteria. The classifications, which have been continued under the reorganization of the NHS, are:

restricted: no additional doctors considered necessary
intermediate: according to circumstances more doctors might or might not be required
open and designate: more doctors required

Financial incentives are given to doctors to set up practices in "designated" areas (Ministry of Health, National Health Services Notes, 2:1). According to Abel-Smith, the secretary of state suggested, in negotiations with the medical profession in 1975, some positive incentives such as special vacations and special rewards. These incentives involved the development of "distinction awards," which would have been given to doctors working in unpopular specialties and areas, and to doctors doing work particularly important to the administration of the NHS. But the negotiations broke down.

The grouping of hospitals for management purposes in the National Health Service brought together different hospital units serving the same population and made it possible to rationalize the distribution of specialists and junior doctors. These improvements could be achieved principally because the NHS was the single employer for all the different professions. During the first decade of the National Health Service (1948–1958), great improvements were made through the training and recruiting of a considerably enlarged staff and through a wider deployment of specialized medical and technical staff (Godber 1975, p. 28). Nevertheless, the supply of physicians has created considerable difficulties in the running of the NHS. Two years before the 1946 NHS Act came into effect, the government set up three committees, under the chairmanship of Sir William Spens, to report on what ought to be the range of incomes of general practitioners, general dental practitioners, consultants, and specialists in the new service. The Committee on Consultants and Specialists also made recommendations about the pay of specialists in training, dividing them into three grades: senior house officers, registrars, and senior registrars. This last grade was intended to provide new advanced training posts in all specialties to give progressive experience and responsibility to candidates hoping ultimately for consultant posts. But it was assumed that those senior registrars who failed in the competition for consultant posts would simply find a place in general practice (Godber 1975, p. 29). This assumption was a first mistake. Indeed, what was really happening by 1950 was that time-expired senior registrars were unable to get consultant jobs and were unwilling to go into general practice. The Ministry of Health tried to deal with this situation by requiring hospital authorities to discontinue the employment of time-expired registrars and senior registrars who had failed to secure higher posts. However, angry reactions from the medical profession forced the hospital authorities to increase the tenure of senior registrars from three to four years and to allow time-expired senior registrars to be retained on a year-to-year basis while they looked for a job. The minstry's measures eased the situation, but did not resolve it. The medical staffing structure in the hospital service was clearly out of balance.

So, in 1955, the now famous Willink Committee was set up "to estimate, on a long-term basis and with due regard to all relevant considerations, the number of medical practitioners likely to be engaged in all branches of the profession in the future and the consequential intake of medical students required." The committee's report did not take sufficiently into account the deficiencies of official statistics, the emigration of doctors dissatisfied with conditions in the NHS to North America and other developed countries, population trends, and developments in medical practice and technology that called for more junior staff. Summing up, the committee declared that, while British medical schools had not produced too many doctors in the past, they soon would do so, and the annual intake of medical students should therefore be reduced by 10 percent (Watkin 1975, p. 225). By 1961 it became sufficiently clear that in this recommendation the Willink Committee had made a serious miscalculation, and throughout the sixties its effects were felt in the serious shortage of junior medical staff. The "competitive apprenticeship staff structure in the hospital specialties" (Godber 1975, p. 29) had still further disastrous consequences. It ensured that medical education was mostly geared to specialist hospital practice and, as a general rule, neither prepared young doctors for work in the community nor stimulated their interest in it (Brown 1973, p. 52). One of the possible ways out of this impasse, advocated by the Royal Commission on Medical Education (Todd Report, 1968), was to reorient the basic training of a doctor, putting more emphasis on primary care, including the social aspects of disease, so that more medical students would become interested in general practice and see it as a worthwhile vocation (Brown 1973, p. 53). The Todd Report further indicated a need to more than double the intake of medical schools (from 2,430 to 5,000) by 1990, by increasing the size of existing schools and by creating new ones (Watkin 1975, p. 250). In 1976 the government placed a very high priority on reaching a yearly student intake of some 4,000 to enable a higher proportion of posts to be filled by British graduates by 1980 (Department of Health and Social Security 1976, p. 15). Another possible way out was to make general practice more attractive by modeling it on hospital practice. This model is consistent with the introduction of the health center concept. On this subject, the Davis Committee was set up "to review the working and organization of group practice, with particular reference to health centers and to make recommendations" (Watkin 1975, p. 259).

Nursing Personnel

Shortages in qualified personnel have similarly had a significant influence on the NHS policy on nursing. The availability of nurses closely reflects demographic changes and the health service's capacity to retain nurses after qualification. Therefore, nurse training has attracted many overseas students and will continue to do so. Further, training schools are showing an increasing readiness to recruit men. The Royal College of Nursing is trying to improve the status of the profession by raising the educational threshold for entry to nurse training, and it wants to reduce the amount of practical work demanded from trainee nurses by making their training more academic. It has been recognized that it would be almost impossible to recruit more young female students if the traditional pattern were followed; therefore, in 1972, the government set up the Briggs Committee "to review the role of the nurse and the midwife in the hospital and the community, and the education and training required for that role, so that the best use is made of available manpower to meet present needs and the needs of an integrated health service." The committee recommended, among other things, a flexible attitude to recruitment, changes in the internal management of hospitals to permit greater use of part-time staff, and an administrative structure that would allow more rational use of the limited reserve of trained nurses (Brown 1973, p. 49). The *Consultative Document* on priorities (Department of Health and Social Security 1976, p. 15) proposed to retain throughout the country at least the existing level of resources devoted to nurse training, and later on to increase them substantially in order to implement the recommendations of the Briggs Report on nurse training.

Other Health Related Personnel

Immediately after the introduction of the NHS, the "professions supplementary to medicine" were reorganized along lines recommended in 1951 by the Cope Committee, established in 1948 "to consider the supply and demand, training and qualifications of certain medical auxiliaries employed in the NHS" (Watkin 1975, p. 338). The Zuckerman Report, 1968, considered the future organization and development of hospital scientific and technical services in NHS hospitals (Watkin 1975, p. 341), and The McMillan Report, 1973, similarly investigated "the future role of the (remedial) professions in relation to other professions and to the patient, and on the pattern of staffing and training needed to meet this" (Watkin 1975, p. 350).

Managerial Personnel

Before the Reorganization Act of 1973, the development of managers was concentrated in the hospitals. The scientific sophistication of hospital medical practice and the separation of a hospital's service into so many specialties meant that specialist work had to be organized (Godber 1975, p. 40). In 1967, the Cogwheel working party recommended a division system: specialties falling into the same broad medical or surgical categories within a hospital or hospital group should be grouped together to form a division. Each division should carry out recurrent appraisals of the services it provided and should cope with management problems within its clinical field. The Ministry of Health asked hospital authorities to encourage their medical staffs to organize themselves along the lines of the report. As was noted in the Second Report of the Joint Working Party (1972), subsequent progress was uneven, with marked regional variations (Watkin 1975, p. 244). Around the time that the first Cogwheel Report was published, another report appeared, namely, the Salmon Report, 1966, from the Committee on Senior Nursing Staff Structure (Ministry of Health 1966). The Salmon Report introduced the language of management into nursing. Nursing services were reorganized under chief nursing officers for hospital groups, and similar principles were being applied to nursing staff of local authorities. Hospital pharmaceutical services were being reorganized in accordance with the Noel Hall Report (Joseph 1972, p. 34).

One of the intentions of the 1973 Reorganization Act was to develop the principles of Cogwheel and Salmon for implementation within the unified NHS, not only in hospitals and other institutions, but also in the RHA's, the AHA's, and the districts (Department of Health and Social Security 1972a). The district is the operational unit. The medical profession in a given district is organized into two main committees: a Local Medical Committee, consisting of all general practitioners, and a so-called Cogwheel organization, comprising the specialists working in hospitals and representatives of the junior medical hospital staff. Six representatives from each organization meet in a district medical committee, together with representatives of doctors working in the community care services, in research, in medical education, and other areas. In this committee a generally acceptable medical view is formulated and then put before a district management team, consisting of one consultant, one general practitioner, a community physician, a nursing officer, a finance officer, and an administrator. This team is a consensus group; that is, all its decisions must be unanimous. It is the function of this team to reach decisions which are acceptable to all these professions in the reorganized NHS (Chester 1975, p. 13).

In these managerial arrangements, an important function is fulfilled by a new health professional, namely, the community physician; this concept originated in the Hunter Report, 1972, which was intended "to review the functions of the medical administrators in the health services and to make recommendations regarding the provision required for their training" (Department of Health and Social Security 1972b). The community physician's role was described in the white paper: "As specialist in . . . community medicine, their concern will be with assessing need for health services, evaluating the effectiveness of existing services and planning the best use of health resources. Equally, they will concern themselves with developing preventive health services, with the link between the health and the local authority personal, social, public health, and education services, and with providing the medical advice and help which local authorities will need for the administration of those and other services" (Joseph 1972, p. 34). The white paper clearly states that concern for human resources should not be limited to a concern for the health professions, and that the success of the NHS increasingly depends on the quality of a whole range of administrative staff (Joseph 1972, p. 33). Hospital administration has rapidly become acknowledged as an important activity in its own right and not something that can be done by other professionals, such as physicians or nurses, in their spare time (Chester 1970, p. 346). Furthermore, the conviction has begun to spread that hospital administration is not a suitable topic for undergraduates and should be reserved for graduate studies. As a consequence, the first British and also the first European graduate school in hospital administration was organized at the University of Manchester in 1956 under the financial sponsorship of the Ministry of Health (Chester 1970, p. 348).

A further important step in the education of hospital administrators was the report of the Committee of Inquiry into the Recruitment, Training, and Promotion of the Administrative and Clerical Staff in the Hospital Service (the Lycett Green Report, 1963). Hospital administrators frequently complained that hospital administration as a career was scarcely recognized by the general public and that the recruitment of able school and university leavers suffered as a result. The complex structure of the NHS and wide local variations in practice made it difficult to explain to a member of the general public what exactly a hospital administrator did and what exactly he was responsible for. The Lycett Green Report, and to a lesser extent the 1957 Report of Sir Noel Hall on "The Grading Structure of Administrative and Clerical Staff in the Hospital Service," made it a little easier to explain a hospital administrator's career structure. One of the Lycett Green Report's most important proposals was to establish a National Staff Committee, consisting of members and officers of hospital authorities, representatives from universities, and a representative of the Ministry of Health, to oversee the recruitment, training, and management development of hospital administrators and to supervise the arrangements for appointing senior staff.

The two existing schemes of training in hospital administration—the national and the regional schemes—were merged and shortened from two-and-a-half to two years. This scheme consisted of planned practical training interspersed with brief periods—the longest was three months—at a university or at the King's Fund College of Hospital Management. Later changes in the scheme shifted the emphasis still further towards practical experience (Watkin 1975, p. 190).

In 1973, the National Staff Committee and the National Nursing Staff Committee, which represented hospital staff only, were reconstituted on an interim basis, with a wider membership, to meet the needs of an integrated health service. Renamed, respectively, the National Staff Committee for Administrative and Clerical Staff and the National Staff Committee for Nurses and Midwives, these committees have similar purposes—to advise the Secretary of State on policies and procedures for recruitment, training, deployment, and development of staff within the NHS as a whole (Department of Health and Social Security 1974, p. 47). Also during 1973, in preparation for the reorganization of the NHS, the DHSS sponsored an extensive program in "Training for Change." Multidisciplinary courses in the management of integrated health care were offered at eight education centers for senior administrative staff in the major professions from all three branches of the then-existing service. In addition to these courses, special short courses for medical administrators in the hospital and local government services were offered throughout the year at the universities of Manchester, Birmingham, and Wales, and at the London School of Hygiene and Tropical Medicine. Members of the new RHA's and AHA's attended short two-day seminars soon after their appointment, mainly at the centers that had conducted the multidisciplinary courses (Department of Health and Social Security 1974, p. 52).

Professional managerialism is threatened by the prevailing economic crisis: the Secretary of State has already advised health authorities that the creation and filling of any administrative posts and the filling of vacancies should not take place until both the need for a post, relative to the specific job of work, and the real priority of the work have been fully considered (Department of Health and Social Security 1976, p. 12). Education for advancement management has been the subject of a working party established by the Kings Fund, which reported in early 1977 and suggested a special program for senior management education (Working party 1977).

Health Consumers

As of 1977, Great Britain was unique among European countries in mandating consumer involvement in its National Health Service. Between the enactment of national health insurance in 1911 and the creation of the NHS in 1948, there were two familiar roles for consumers in health care. First, lay involvement in health insurance: the 1911 Insurance Act mandated that medical benefits were to be administered in every county by a local insurance committee of forty to eighty members, three-fifths of whom were to be insured persons. Second, voluntary hospitals continued to have distinguished public representatives on their boards.

The 1948 NHS Act abolished the insurance committees. At the same time virtually all hospitals, both voluntary and public, were nationalized. Fifteen Regional Hospital Boards were created. The members of these boards were not to be self-perpetuating (as the voluntary hospital boards had been), but rather were appointed by the minister of health after consultation. Thus, the net effect of the National Health Service was to eliminate the modest local consumer role existing before 1948, by replacing it with greatly increased central government power. The only way in which the consumer could now participate was as a voter or, as a member of a political party, by influencing members of Parliament. To remedy these deficiencies, the 1973 Reorganization Act created two official mechanisms, making the NHS more responsive to the consumer. A Health Service Commissioner for England, Scotland, and Wales was appointed, who, together with his staff, carries out "investigations into complaints concerned with hospitals and other health services." The commissioner cannot inquire into matters related to clinical judgements of a health professional. He cannot contravene judgments of a health professional. He further cannot intervene until the body complained against has been given an opportunity to consider the complaint. During its first eighteen months, the Commissioner's office received 612 complaints. Three hundred and fifty-four were rejected as outside the jurisdiction of the office, 152 were investigated and reports were filed, and 106 were carried further. The commissioner has no power to compel settlement of complaints, but has extraordinary and independent power to investigate. Although the specifics of the cases investigated are kept confidential, the commissioner publishes summaries of the problems dealt with and the way in which they are resolved.

The second new mechanism, the Community Health Council, was brought into being by the 1973 Reorganization Act expressly to introduce greater democratization into the NHS. One CHC is organized for each district management team and there are thus 229 CHC's in England and Wales. Each board is made up exclusively of lay persons (that is, health professionals and NHS employees are excluded). Half the board members are named by local authorities, one-third by voluntary organizations, such as the Red Cross and the Heart Association, and one-sixth by the Area Health Authority. All reports and plans of the district management team and the Area Health Authority must be brought before the local CHC for review and comment before they can take effect. At this time the CHC has no power except to open up the working of the NHS and to develop community pressure, but these are significant tasks. Each CHC has a salaried secretary and there are plans to evolve an appropriate national council for Community Health Councils. The effect of CHC's thus far has been to heighten local consumer consciousness, to develop the expertise of board members, and to force the professionals to begin taking community attitudes into account. In addition to the two structures described above, there are a variety of unofficial local initiatives by and on behalf of consumers. One example is the Disability Alliance, a federation of thirty-seven organizations of disabled individuals constituted in 1974 to bring about more equitable standards of living among the disabled and to ensure them of the fullest opportunity for personal development.

Physical Resources

Hospitals

In the United Kingdom hospitals have developed in widely differing ways. The earliest voluntary hospitals were founded in the middle of the eighth century (monastery infirmaries date from even earlier times). Over the years, a large number of such hospitals or infirmaries were established. Some were to be the main places for the development of medical education and of specialist services. The Poor Law Act of 1835 led to widespread institutional development, including infirmaries, because medical indigence could lead to admission and retention in such an institution (Godber 1975, p. 5).

As already stated, the 1911 National Health Insurance Act did not directly affect the position of the hospitals, apart from the provisions concerning the development of sanatoria and the awarding of grants to voluntary hospitals. "The government had not legislated for the hospitals because they believed in the voluntary system and wanted it to continue. If they legislated for the hospitals they would be bound to a certain amount of government control over their work" (Abel-Smith 1964, p. 241). Grants to voluntary hospitals proved to be of no importance, in contrast to those to sanatoria. Abel-Smith states: "Initially, the Government made available the sum of £1,500,000 for the construction of new accommodation. Local authorities who built sanatoria were granted three-fifths of the cost of approved schemes, local authorities who built tuberculosis dispensaries were given four-fifths of the cost. In the case of insured persons, a sum of £1,000,000 was set aside in the insurance fund to be spent by insurance committees on sanatorium benefits. In the case of the dependents of the insured persons and non-insured persons, local authorities could obtain half the cost of treatment from the Local Government Board" (Abel-Smith 1964, p. 239).

Another trend in the evolution of the British hospital system was the growing legal responsibility of the local authorities before World War II. For instance, in 1920 the National Insurance Act was amended and sanatorium benefits were removed from the scheme by making the provision of inpatient care for all tuberculosis cases the responsibility of the county and the county borough councils. However, many councils made grants to voluntary hospitals to provide care instead of creating their own sanatoria (Abel-Smith 1964, p. 294).

From 1920 onwards, local authorities also had the responsibility for providing maternity services. But local-authority maternity units were often separate and too small, or they were converted blocks in what had been Poor Law infirmaries (Godber 1975, p. 9). A new opportunity to challenge the supremacy of the voluntary hospitals—if one wished to do so—was given the local authorities by the Local Government Act, 1929. This act handed over the hospital functions of the Poor Law to the local authorities, although each authority was free to decide to what extent accommodation for the sick would no longer be provided under the Poor Law and instead would be run as part of the general public health services (Abel-Smith 1964, p. 368). In general, then, "while some authorities were attempting to provide a service to the public, there were others who made little progress in their health services" (Abel-Smith 1964, p. 383).

Most of the local authorities were too small and too poor to provide an adequate hospital service. The standards achieved by some authorities—particularly the largely rural authorities—left much to be desired. And the local authorities' boundaries did not facilitate planning, since urban areas and the surrounding county were often controlled by different authorities. This led to different plans for joint authorities. Similarly, the white paper of 1944 advised that hospitals should be the responsibility of joint authorities, which would take over and run all local-authority hospitals. However, all such plans proved to be unacceptable to the doctors, who showed an intense dislike of local government and its control over part of the hospital system (Willcocks 1967, p. 63).

In the meantime, the voluntary sector was also actively developing hospital resources. "In 1921 the proportion of patients being treated in voluntary hospitals was about 25 percent: by 1938 this proportion had risen to 36 percent. The role of the public sector dropped from 75 percent of the patients to 64 percent. While a spectacular expansion of accommodation was under way in the voluntary sector, there was hardly any increase in the number of beds provided in the public sector . . . It is not surprising therefore that throughout the inter-war period most of these who worked in the voluntary hospitals believed that the voluntary movement had an indefinite future" (Abel-Smith 1964, p. 385). Up to 1944, there had still been no serious talks about abolishing the voluntary hospital "system." Willcocks states: "one feature of the White Paper that received welcome from all medical and hospital groups was the continuation of the dual hospital system of voluntary and local authority hospitals" (Willcocks 1967, p. 64). Instead of abolishing the voluntary hospitals, the 1944 white paper proposed that those voluntary hospitals willing to participate in the scheme would have to accept the area plan to be drawn up by the joint authorities. The day-to-day running of the hospitals, however, would be left to the voluntary hospitals' governing bodies. Thus, neither for the local-authority hospitals nor for the voluntary hospitals did this white paper propose the radical changes that were subsequently judged necessary, including, in particular, changes in hospital ownership.

It was Aneurin Bevan who came to the vital conclusion "that the ownership of all the hospitals, whether they were owned by local authorities or voluntary hospitals, was to be transferred to the Minister of Health" (Godber 1975, p. 16). Only three years earlier, hardly anyone had been prepared to advocate such an extreme solution to the problems of hospital planning and administration. But on July 5, 1948, most of Britain's hospitals were taken into national ownership.

Why were all the solutions proposed earlier rejected? Abel-Smith states: "The pressure which led to this development came not from any doctrines of the Labor Party, which by 1945 was confining its proposals for nationalization to the industrial sector, but from the aspiration of parts of the medical profession. Nationalization seemed the only way by which the consultants and specialists could achieve their principal objectives: adequate financial support for the hospital in which they worked, the retention of private practice and an effective 'say' in the running of all hospital services" (Abel-Smith 1964, p. 488). Titmuss suggests similar reasons. Examining the rejection of the alternative to common ownership, namely a contractual relationship with the voluntary hospitals, Titmuss concluded that if the government limited its responsibilities to a contractual relationship, such an arrangement would still leave the majority of doctors as salaried employees of the municipal authorities, while many members of the profession, having had some actual experience of the state-run EMS, preferred a centrally controlled organization. The profession made it abundantly clear that it would enter the service only on condition that all the hospitals were taken out of the hands of municipal governments (Titmuss 1958, p. 141).

Thus, from 1948 on, the hospitals became a complete responsibility of the central government and as a result had to compete for funds with other government responsibilities such as factories, houses, and schools. According to Abel-Smith, since World War II, half of Britain's schools, nearly half of Britain's houses, but only a quarter of Britain's hospitals have been rebuilt or renovated by the government; these facts reveal clearly the order of government priorities.

After the establishment of the NHS in 1948, there was soon severe criticism that "this public enterprise was failing," "costs were getting out of control," "it was over-centralized," and so forth (Titmuss 1958, p. 148). In 1953, the Conservative government then in office set up the Gillebaud Committee to review "the present and prospective cost of the NHS." The committee reported in 1956. "What was expected was a strong recommendation for economy. Instead, there were recommendations for spending, especially capital expenditure on hospitals and welfare provisions for old people" (Titmuss 1958, p. 149). In the recommendations on the hospital service, the committee suggested that some of the Ministry controls on capital expenditure and staff establishment should be eased (Watkin 1975, p. 145). Few years later, a BMA document demanded a rate of capital investment in hospitals of £50 million a year, where only £100 million had been spent in the entire first decade of the NHS, and that mainly for maintenance (Godber 1975, p. 34).

In 1962, the first comprehensive blueprint for modernizing the hospital service appeared (Ministry of Health 1962). During 1961, all regions had been asked to produce plans, from which this first hospital building plan for the country was assembled. It was followed a year later by a health and welfare services plan. According to Sir George Godber, these plans "mark the end of the period of patching and making do and the first reasoned attempt to go forward on the national scales required" (Godber 1975, p. 34).

At first sight, the idea of reducing the ratio of beds to population, proposed by the Hospital Plan of 1962, seems surprising. But the reason for this proposal was that the number of beds had come to be regarded as less important than their effective utilization: it was thought that streamlining the system would be more efficient than providing large numbers of expensive extra beds. In the 1962 plan, the key element in British hospital planning was the district general hospital of 600 to 800 beds, providing specialist care for all but the rarest forms of illness (patients with these illnesses are sent to a regional center) for a population of 100,000 to 150,000.

The first official review of the district general hospital concept came in 1969 with the report of the Bonham-Carter Committee. This committee recommended much larger district general hospitals, each serving a population of 200,000 or, in the larger cities and conurbations, a population of 300,000. This meant hospitals of 1,000–1,750 beds. On the other hand, the committee's recommendations on the organization of the hospital service assumed a corresponding development of the community services, both in quality and quantity (Watkin 1975, p. 160). But the report was accorded a rather lukewarm reception by the government. It was argued that the new proposals subordinated the convenience and the welfare of patients to the effectiveness of the medical and technological machine. Therefore, the secretary of state, Keith Joseph, decided to retain smaller community hospitals. Since then, there has been a clear shift from the district general hospital concept of planning to the concept of district health services organization—that is, the provision in every district of an integrated complex of comprehensive general hospitals and health centers or group practices. The DHSS's circular of March 1975 (DS 85/75) recommends a pattern of hospital services that includes, first, a district general hospital, providing for the whole population of its district a full range of specialized treatment, and, second, community hospitals, for those patients not requiring the full specialist facilities of a district general hospital. The DHSS is developing a design for a small hospital of about 300 beds, called the nucleus hospital. It will provide a range of standard departments that can be selected to suit local needs. It will be capable of subsequent expansion from the original nucleus to a hospital in the range of 600 to 900 beds (Department of Health and Social Security 1976, p. 23). The 1976 *Consultative Document* on priorities (Department of Health and Social Security 1976) envisages a level of growth for general and acute hospital services which is considerably less than in recent years (½ percent a year in the future, as against 4 percent now). The main part of this small increase will be for geriatric and psychiatric services.

The existence of private patient beds in NHS hospitals has always aroused some controversy. The 1946 NHS Act set aside a number of beds for private patients in NHS hospitals (Section 5 of the 1946 Act). This provision was subsequently replaced by Section 1 of the Health Service and Public Health Act, 1968, which provided that any beds within the total the hospital was allowed by the secretary of state could be used for private patients, instead of just those beds specifically designated for private patients, as previously. The Labor government of Prime Minister James Callaghan has announced its intention to abolish the use of NHS facilities for private purposes altogether. Its proposals are embodied in the Health Services Act of November 22, 1976. This act is intended to secure "the progressive withdrawal of accomodation and services at NHS hospitals from use in connection with the treatment of persons at such hospitals as resident or non-resident private patients" (Section 2,1). Section 3 requires the secretary of state, within six months of the passing of the act (that is, by May 21, 1977), to reduce by 1,000 the total number of beds available for resident private patients, and to ensure that as far as practicable these 1,000 beds are made available to NHS patients. Section 1 establishes the Health Services Board, comprising two doctors, two trade union officials, and a lawyer chairman. It is the duty of the board to submit proposals for the progressive withdrawal of facilities for private patients in NHS hospitals to the secretary of state from time to time, and it is the duty of the secretary of state to give effect to all the proposals submitted. The provisions relate to facilities for outpatient consultants and to therapeutic and diagnostic services, as well as to inpatient beds. The act also aims to control hospital building outside the NHS. No one may construct or extend so-called controlled premises without the authorization of the Health Services Board. Controlled premises, according to the act, are hospitals or nursing homes that are not crown property, that provide facilities for one or more of the following: surgery under general anesthesia; obstetrics; radiotherapy; renal dialysis, radiology, or diagnostic pathology; and that provide 75 or more beds (100 or more in Greater London). As a consequence of this act, most private hospitals to be established in the future are thought likely to contain less than 75 beds (100 in Greater London) (The Health Services Act 1976).

Health Centers

Health Centers, as group practices of primary care physicians, have developed very slowly in Great Britain. Concern about the unexpectedly high costs of the NHS in its early years made successive ministers unwilling to grant the money necessary for the local authorities to build health centers; thus, according to Abel-Smith, health centers were actively discouraged in the beginning. The medical profession itself objected to health centers. Moreover, apart from professional satisfaction, there were no incentives for the general practitioner to improve his surgery or to employ auxiliary staff: "Owing to a curious system of pooling practice expenses, the general practitioner who paid for better equipment and the rent for adequate premises did so, in effect, at his own expense and ended up worse off than his less conscientious colleague" (Brown 1973, p. 37).

Since 1966, general practitioners have been reimbursed for the greater part of their rent and have received financial inducements to work from shared premises. The new financial arrangements paved the way to a revival of interest in health centers. Interest in health centers has accelerated, moreover, for two other reasons. First, the rising cost of land and building has made it more difficult for general practitioners to find suitable accommodations privately. Second, legislative changes and changes in medical opinion have made it possible for community nursing staff to work in group practice centers under the direct control of general practitioners, so that a general practitioner can have the same sort of nursing support in the community that his specialist counterpart has long taken for granted in the hospital (Brown 1973, p. 37). Finally, as a result of the policy of encouraging the provision of health centers, local authorities are no longer allowed to build new clinics for mothers and young children without at the same time making provision for additional services on the health center model. This created an extra impetus for the development of health centers (Brown 1973, p. 39).

In 1973, 104 new health centers were opened, bringing the total number in operation to 468. A three months' pause in new public building, imposed by the government in October 1973, resulted in the postponement of some construction plans, although at the end of that year 148 health centers were being built (Department of Health and Social Security 1974, p. 28). Recent developments have included a considerable increase in the last five years in the number of health centers: only 124 were opened between 1948 and 1969, but since then there have been a further 453, and about 15 percent of all general practitioners now practice from them (Department of Health and Social Security 1976, p. 17). One of the emphases of the 1976 *Consultative Document* on priorities is a further development of health centers. In spite of the general need to reduce capital expenditure, a substantial program is proposed, and priority has been given to the establishment of health centers in areas where inadequate accommodation is hampering the development of primary care teams (Department of Health and Social Security 1976, p. 18).

Information Resources

Health Research

In England and Wales research has been regarded as a national resource, subject to government scrutiny, since the turn of the century. Health research has been a forerunner in this respect. In 1918, the Haldane Report on the *Machinery of Government* stressed the importance of research findings for national policy, that is, to promote the health of the entire country. Though it could not predict in which direction research would progress, this report anticipated a "Department of Intelligence" with its own minister.

Since 1919, university grants have been administered by an independent committee that receives a block allocation from the Treasury to be distributed among the universities according to the committee's judgment of their needs. This committee is the University Grants Committee, and it acts as a buffer between the universities and the central government authorities. While the existence of a buffer has advantages, it also renders the dialogue between the political authorities and the scientific community more difficult. This leads to the danger that research may not be geared to the needs of the population at all.

In 1911, the National Health Insurance Act stated that "the Insurance Commissioners may retain the whole or any part of the sums so payable out of moneys provided by Parliament—one penny per insured person for sanatorium benefits—to be applied, in accordance with regulations made by the Commissioners, for the purposes of research" (Section 16). Though this measure was not mandatory, there was no doubt that it would be carried out. In due course it yielded approximately £51,000 per annum, dispensed, through executive decision, not by the county or county borough-based insurance committees but by a single research organization: the Medical Research Committee, which was subsequently incorporated in 1920 under its present title, the Medical Research Council.

At present, government funds for health research are channeled through either the University Grants Committee, the Medical Research Council, or, since the 1946 National Health Service Act, the Department of Health, later the Department of Health and Social Security. These government funds are supplemented by public money obtained through direct subscription, for example, the British Empire Cancer Campaign and the Imperial Cancer Research Fund; by funds from private foundations such as the Wellcome Trust and the Nuffield Provincial Hospitals Trust; and by funds from industry, such as the National Coal Board and the pharmaceutical industry. From the start, the impact of such an institution as the Nuffield Provincial Hospitals Trust in directing health services research, either through initial funds for pioneer research projects or by influencing a research policy, far exceeded the relative size of its funds involved. It has been stated that "whenever the private foundations provided stimulus or support, the caliber of the research efforts was generally superior . . . It is one of the firmer impressions that private and public support of research and of innovations in health services still fruitfully complement one another, even in the twentieth year of the National Health Service" (Bierman et al. 1968, p. 78).

Medical research is mostly conducted in the universities, the teaching hospitals associated with the twenty-nine existing university-based medical schools, and in the university-affiliated research institutes. The professionals in charge of teaching are expected to engage in research, while many researchers also carry teaching functions. Some 10 percent (Organization for Economic Cooperation and Development 1972, p. 4) of the general university funds are drawn in the form of grants from the University Grants Committee (UGC). Since its creation in 1919, its function has never been challenged. Acting as the intermediary between the central authorities and the universities, the UGC allocates block grants with no strings attached to guarantee a sufficient income for teaching and research staff (the UGC regards teaching and research as complementary functions). Earmarked funds only represent a small proportion of the total UGC budget. Though the UGC sometimes suggests specific purposes for certain budget allocations, it invariably adds that these suggestions are not binding. The grants are allotted on a five-year basis, after which the universities' budget requirements are reviewed for the next five-year period. However, in itself the system remains flexible: supplementary grants may be made within the five-year period, while the university is not obliged to spend one-fifth of the total allocation each year.

Until 1962, the grant allocation mechanism was rather static, depending primarily on criteria such as the number of students projected, student/teacher ratios, floor space per student. After 1962, the committee began to get involved in the elaboration of a policy to coordinate university development. In view of university expansion plans and restrained government resources, it had to assume responsibility for balancing teaching and research, as well as different studies and courses. A 1962 "Memorandum of General Guidance" expresses views on the development of seven disciplines, including dentistry, but nevertheless states that "the Committee hopes that universities will find it helpful to have the considerations mentioned in this memorandum before them when they come to decide their own development policies and priorities for the quinquennium" (Organization for Economic Cooperation and Development 1972, p. 91).

The Medical Research Council (MRC), established in 1920 under royal charter as an independent body with considerable autonomy, responsible to the secretary of state for education and science, is one of the five research councils that provide supplementary research funds in selected fields based on criteria of scientific quality and national importance. The MRC is the most progressive attempt we found, in the five countries studied, to reconcile mission-oriented research with the undifferentiated financing of fundamental research, though some critics feel that this reconciliation occurs at the expense of mission-oriented research (Organization for Economic Cooperation and Development 1972, p. 46). Its twelve to sixteen members are all appointed by the secretary of state, and no fewer than three-quarters of them are appointed on the basis of their scientific qualifications, which are determined in consultation with the Royal Society. To plan and carry out its research program, the council has three advisory boards: the Clinical Research Board, set up in 1953 in consultation with the Ministry of Health to assist in developing clinical research in the NHS; the Biological Research Board; and the Tropical Medicine Research Board.

In recent years the council has tried to play a more dynamic role, rather than simply reacting passively to proposals emanating from the universities. A set of specialized scientific committees has been established to explore possibilities in new fields and to follow up on developments, where necessary: as of 1972, there were four research grants committees, six working groups, and twenty subcommittees and round tables, most of which were problem-oriented. The MRC supports and subsidizes medical research in three main ways.

First, the MRC employs a large scientific and technical staff who work either in the council's own research establishments (as of 1973 these include three large establishments: the National Institute for Medical Research, the Laboratory of Molecular Biology, and the Clinical Research Center), or, as of 1972, in over seventy smaller research units, which are normally attached to universities and hospitals and are formed around a single distinguished research worker; some of these small units are abroad. As of January 1, 1972, there were 1,099 scientific staff, of whom 321 were medically qualified, and 1,690 were technical staff (Central Office of Information 1973, p. 50). This research-unit mechanism was initiated in 1960 when the council reviewed its policy in order to accelerate research in universities where long-term plans were found to coincide with national needs in the council's field of interest. Each university selected was given a grant to enlarge its research staff and facilities and in return agreed to take over the entire financial responsibility for the research project after a certain lapse of time, usually five or seven years. Over the period 1962–1972, no such units were disbanded while thirty-five new ones were created.

Second, the council makes grants to independent workers for short-term research projects, mainly in universities and hospitals, but occasionally also to private institutions, such as the Institute of Cancer Research. Third, the council awards a number of fellowships, scholarships, and travelling fellowships.

The MRC's policy of financing research units concentrated around a single distinguished research worker results in a proliferation of independent and sometimes overlapping research projects. Indeed, until now the MRC has not been very successful in launching cooperative research projects nor in formulating a coherent higher education policy in cooperation with the UGC. Research project effectiveness has thus suffered a little because of the policy of research independence. However, corrective action is under way. In 1964, the government announced its commitment to applied research. This interest, together with the tendency of many independent research units to become highly specialized over the years, may indeed bring about unavoidably, though indirectly, a recognition of the need for cooperation. This trend has been reenforced by two recent developments: first, the establishment of the MRC's Clinical Research Center, commissioned in 1960 and inaugurated in 1970; and second, a shift in research fund dispensing capability from the Medical Research Council to the DHSS, a change decided upon in 1972.

The Department of Health and Social Security (from 1919 to 1969, the Ministry of Health) has been interested and involved in research since its very beginning. Much of its early work concerned the control of communicable diseases and sanitary conditions. Even though the NHS Act of 1946 contained a clause stating that the "Minister may conduct or assist by grants or otherwise any person to conduct research into any matter relating to the causation, prevention, diagnosis or treatment of illness or mental defectiveness," until 1963–64, the department's research interests were limited to the Public Health Laboratory Service, and, following agreement with the MRC in 1958–59, a scheme of grants for minor hospital-organized research projects, run either through the regional hospital boards or through the ministry itself. Criticism, however, was already mounting. A distinction emerged between the concepts of the DHSS as a commercial organization providing incentives to innovation and improvement and as a civil service department adjusting to the status quo rather than planning development for the future (Cohen 1971, p. 6). As a result of the 1956 Guillebaud Committee of Inquiry into the Costs of the NHS, the department began to change, with the Nuffield Provincial Hospitals Trust acting as the main catalyst for health services involvement. Methods of producing and using statistical indexes and other measures of efficiency were developed, as were hospital building programs, including relevant standards, equipmént and supplies, organization and methods, and the definition of standards of good practice in hospitals.

In 1960 the whole area of clinical research also came under review, and in 1963–64 the DHSS approved the allocation of funds for operational research work in the broadest sense. Two years later, similar funds were allotted to support research and development in building and engineering of health facilities. In 1964, the general practitioners and local health and welfare services became the special focus of health services research. In 1966–67, the department reviewed its activities, and as a result set up a Medical Research Branch and a Statistics and Research Division. All along, the DHSS's relations with the MRC have been cordial, because of the personalities involved, and an increasingly cooperative and coordinated research effort has developed, which was enhanced by the inauguration of the Clinical Research Center at Northwick Park Hospital in 1970.

The DHSS research efforts are primarily extramural and involve university or medical school departments, local government establishments, and NHS hospitals or service departments. Topics include medical, social, and operational research, service development research, and research and development on supplies and appliances (McLachlan 1971, 1973).

The rapid expansion of DHSS research activities continued throughout the sixties, and by 1971 NHS research was seriously under way. Some advocated the need for a Health Services Research Council—since the Social Service Research Council founded in 1965 was not concerned with the health services—but NHS reorganization and the publication of the Rothschild Committee green paper on "A Framework for Government Research and Development" in November 1971, and the government's white paper on the same subject in July 1972, encouraged another approach. The customer/contractor principle was finally endorsed, a transfer of funds from the research councils to the executive departments—some 25 percent of the funds in the case of the MRC—was advocated, and the position of chief scientist was introduced within the executive departments as the basis of new developments. These three principles have since been worked out in greater detail and have resulted in a more systematic and coordinated approach to medical research-and-development policy both within and without the DHSS; the links between the DHSS and the Medical Research Council, and, to a lesser extent, the Social Services Research Council, have been strengthened. For 1970–71, government expenditure on health research can be estimated at £51.5 million, of which almost £20.0 million was dispensed by the University Grants Committee, some £21 million by the Medical Research Council, and some £5.6 million by the DHSS (Central Office of Information 1973, p. 48).

Health Statistics

The Medical Act of 1858 established the General Medical Council as the first registering body to keep track of competent and qualified physicians (Central Office of Information 1973, p. 55). The 1911 National Health Insurance Act specified in Section 60 the duty of the insurance committees "to make reports as to the health of insured persons and to furnish statistical and other returns." Nevertheless, the pragmatic results of this section were not as extensive as its wording may imply. The first impetus towards the development of a health information system resulted from the circumstances that led to World War II. The state became more actively interested in its able-bodied population for defense and war production purposes, and this led to a renewed interest in vital statistics and population censuses. Then, when the Emergency Medical Service was organized in 1938 the Ministry of Health decided to hold its first official survey of hospitals and their running conditions in Britain, with the help of the Nuffield Trust (Ministry of Health *National Health Services Notes,* 12:1). Though the results were instrumental in the creation of a National Health Service after the war, nevertheless, the NHS paid limited attention during its first years to the question of further health information systems. Although the very creation of the NHS theoretically removed most organizational constraints on health information systems, little was done within the NHS—except for the collection of common statistics such as number of beds and inpatients—to develop a coherent set of health information parameters that would improve its efficiency and effectiveness.

The NHS Act of 1948 stipulated that each hospital should prepare annual cost returns in a form prescribed by the ministry, which resulted in a uniform accounting scheme known as the hospital costing returns. However, little comparative analysis was done initially, and the actual influence of this scheme on policy was difficult to pinpoint. The cost data were linked neither to production data nor to hospital activity data. In contrast, epidemiological research, with well-defined population and patient samples, developed extensively and allowed for the testing of hypotheses on ecological and personal factors and their relation to the population's health problems. The development of health information systems began to improve at the beginning of the sixties, after the publication of the Guillebaud Committee's report on the costs of the NHS in 1956. A central intelligence unit began to emerge. An Advisory Committee for Management Efficiency was given responsibility to coordinate all studies on hospitals under the auspices of the executive secretary's office. One-third of these studies were sponsored by the Ministry of Health itself, one-third by philanthropic organizations such as the Nuffield Provincial Hospitals Trust, and the remaining third by regional hospital boards or universities. The DHSS's Statistical Branch was also reinforced at that time and launched a 10 percent random sampling of hospital inpatients ("Hospital Inpatient Enquiry," or HIPE), which was subsequently replaced by a more sophisticated hospital activity analysis. Many similar initiatives resulted in classic studies such as Forsyth and Logan's investigation of hospital utilization in a geographically and medically isolated population of 11,600 (Forsyth and Logan 1960) and Barr's work at the Operations Research Group of the Oxford Regional Hospital Board.

At present, special surveys on many types of NHS activities are abundant, though coherence, record linkage, and streamlining of the different data banks still seems to be lacking. This lack of coherence appears to have two causes: the relatively short-term financial basis on which most of the experimental work (prerequisite for ongoing data collection) must be done, and the lack of trained professionals to develop these information resources and to use them for managerial purposes. The confidential character of these health information systems also certainly acted, till recently, as a braking power. Manpower statistics were for a long time underdeveloped, despite the enormous problems that the NHS encounters in matching supply and demand. Although the 1946 NHS Act suggested that the executive committees should report to the Medical Practices Committee on the number of general practitioners required, the occurrence of vacancies, and the need to fill such vacancies, this management instrument never evolved into a comprehensive health manpower information system. This lack was exposed most dramatically when, in 1957, the Willink Report announced a coming surplus of physicians, a position that had to be reversed within a few years. The 1973 Reorganization Act, and in particular the annual NHS planning cycle that resulted from it, provided a new impetus for the comprehensive health management information system that has slowly begun to emerge.

In Retrospect

The case of England and Wales is special among the five countries studied. They decided after World War II to abandon contributory health insurance as the main national effort and replace it with direct provision of health care by the government. The country thus became the model of the welfare state. More than is generally realized, the NHS came into being by a unique combination of wartime conditions, medical politics, economic constraints, and a basic commitment—which grew out of the war—toward building a new and more egalitarian society. At the start the NHS simply nationalized and consolidated the prevailing health care delivery system. Eventually, through the 1973 Reorganization Act, the system became fully integrated.

4 | France

In 1930, after a decade of proposals and an approved, but never implemented, act of 1928, the French health insurance scheme started as part of a comprehensive social security plan. The plan has not been changed fundamentally since then. The postwar period witnessed an extension of the coverage to every citizen and attempts to simplify the administrative machinery. Faced with a strongly organized and militant medical profession, the French national health program has mainly been preoccupied, apart from extending the insurance coverage, with hospital affairs. The hospital legislation of 1958 focused on the public hospital, and the reform of 1970 embraced all types of hospitals.

1930: A Modest Start Toward Comprehensive Health Insurance

In 1920, the French minister of labor, Jourdain, established a committee to draft a social insurance bill, including health insurance. Introduced to the House of Representatives in 1921 by Grinda, this bill was unanimously approved, after major changes by the House, in 1924. After the elections of that year, the bill was transmitted to the Senate, where it was approved in 1927, but only after being entirely revised. The House agreed to the new text in 1928, once again just before the elections. This approved bill became the Act on Social Insurance, passed on April 5, 1928 (Loi du 5 avril 1928). However, this act was never implemented. It was only a "preelectoral manifestation," intended to win votes in the 1928 election. It was merely a declaration of principles, and both government and Parliament tacitly agreed that the bill, when approved, would never be executed (Hatz-feld 1963, p. 40). Moreover, the opposition of trade unions, employers, physicians, landlords, and farm workers inhibited the promulgation of the needed statutory regulations (Dupeyroux 1975, p. 55). After different proposals and amendments passed back and forth between the House and Senate, in 1930 a bill amending the 1928 Act was finally approved. It became the 1930 Act Amending and Completing the 1928 Act on Social Insurance (Loi du 30 avril 1930). Although this 1930 act was called an amendment, it actually revised completely the 1928 act, and it remains up to now the basis of the French social security scheme (Van Langendonck 1971, p. 63).

A Confrontation of Principles

One of the forces in favor of health insurance was organized labor. Following World War I, the working classes had gained political power, resulting in successive electoral victories. Organized labor became an important lobby and a driving force behind the introduction of compulsory health insurance. More leftist labor organizations, however, rejected social insurance, because they saw it as democratic bluff or because they were against compulsory employee contributions, which was also the objection of the Communist party (Jambu-Merlin 1970, p. 23). Compulsory social insurance was supported by the civil servants, because they considered the execution of compulsory insurance an extension of their function that would finally give them greater recognition and prestige (Hatzfeld 1971, p. 31).

The medical profession proved to be a serious opponent to compulsory health insurance. In 1927, French physicians formulated and adopted their famous Medical Charter, propounding four basic principles that the profession believed should be respected in the relation between physicians and the health insurance funds: (1) the patient must be free to choose his physician; (2) the physician must be free to prescribe drugs and medicines; (3) the physician and patient must be allowed to bargain directly over the fee; and (4) professional secrecy must be respected. These four principles were clearly a reaction against the 1921 proposal, which had called for collective agreements between the funds and the medical profession and stipulated that the physicians would be paid on the basis of an annual fee per capita through the cooperation of the medical unions, as was the practice in Germany at the time (Hatzfeld 1963, p. 41). The 1928 act had already replaced the per capita fee system with a system of payment on a fee-for-service basis (this meant an important victory for the physicians), but had not indicated clearly whether the physicians would be paid by the funds or by the patients. In the end, the 1930 act was a complete victory for the medical profession, because the Medical Charter was integrated into the act (Galant 1955, p. 14).

Employers opposed compulsory social insurance as being at variance with the laissez-faire doctrine then still accepted. Small employers, especially, regarded the obligation to pay social insurance contributions as a real danger to their survival. Originally, farm workers and their employers opposed the idea of compulsory insurance, but they finally gave in because the 1930 act assured them the same advantages as other workers while they only had to pay one-quarter of the normal contributions (Henry 1930).

Scope and Content of the 1930 Act

Coverage. The 1930 act made a distinction between compulsory insurance and voluntary insurance. All wage earners employed in industry and commerce who were not older than sixty years and earned less than 15,000 francs per year were compulsorily insured. Voluntary insurance was open to farmers, market gardeners, small employers and white collar workers, earning not more than 15,000 francs per year. The insured's wife and his children below sixteen years were also covered.

Financing. Under the 1930 act, social insurance was financed partly by contributions made by employers and employees, partly by a state subsidy, and partly by copayments. The employer had to pay the sum of his contribution and that of the employee, but he could deduct one-half from the worker's salary. The state's subsidy varied yearly, according to the excess of costs over contributions. Because farm workers and their employers only paid one-quarter of the normal contributions, in the beginning years this state subsidy was already very high. Charges to patients covered 15–20 percent of the total costs.

Benefits. Health insurance covered the costs of general practitioner and specialist treatment, drugs and appliances, hospitalization and treatment in health care institutions, and surgical treatment and dental prostheses that had been approved by a technical committee. Waiting periods for payment of these benefits varied between 60 and 240 days. Moreover, the benefits were only provided for a maximum of six months for any one episode of illness.

Health insurance was generally administered by the primary funds. These were the mutual societies that had developed in the nineteenth century from widely different sources, including labor unions, employers' organizations, and parishes. The insured were free to choose any primary fund. The departmental and interdepartmental primary funds (the "department" in France is equivalent to a province elsewhere) served those insured who had not chosen to join a local primary fund. To function as primary funds, mutual societies had to be recognized by the minister of labor. The funds negotiated agreements with the medical unions, but as a consequence of the medical profession's severe opposition to the general idea of compulsory health insurance, agreements on fees were only binding to the funds and not to the physicians. These agreements were subject to the approval of a departmental committee, whose members were one-third fund representatives, one-third physician representatives, and one-third representatives of the ministries of Labor and Public Health, including hospital representatives.

Health Resources Development in the 1930 Act

Two articles of the 1930 act provided for the development of physical resources for health care.

1. Article 28.3 stated that the primary funds could cooperate to realize so-called public utility projects such as health care institutions, preventive care institutions, sanatoriums, nursing homes, and convalescent homes.
2. Article 33.4 stated that the insurance funds could use their accumulated assets to create or develop such institutions as mentioned in Article 28.3.

The act even included provision for an embryonic planning system: Article 29 empowered the funds to use their disposable money to acquire land or buildings, such as hospitals or other health care institutions; but, in cities where a medical school already existed, such institutions could only be built after the advice of the local hospital administrative committee and the medical school board. Interestingly, the funds were explicitly forbidden to establish pharmacies.

Neither the originators nor the precise results of these articles have been discovered. Even before 1930, a few health care institutions had been created through the support of the mutual societies. There are no data available to prove that the specific provisions of the 1930 act allowing the mutual societies to create health care institutions had any appreciable impact.

1958: Hospital Reforms, A First Round

The Driving Forces

Immediately after World War II, the French felt a need to reorganize and simplify the social security system (attempts had already been made in this direction before the war, in 1935, and during the war, in 1941 and 1942). This reorganization was given legal expression through Regulation 45-2250 of October 5, 1945. In this regulation, the multiple funds and societies were replaced by one official fund per department (departmental funds). In some cases there were also official funds for smaller administrative units: primary funds and regional funds. At the national level a national social security fund was established. This reorganization actually meant that, in the administration of compulsory health insurance, the mutual societies were replaced by public- and state-controlled bodies. But the mutual societies were not abolished completely, since they continued to administer the complementary schemes. This attempt to simplify the administrative organization was not very successful, however, and eventually Regulation 67-706 of August 21, 1967, introduced yet another new administrative structure.

The social security system (including health insurance) was considerably extended by Regulation 45-2454 of October 19, 1945. During the postwar decades, this extension was implemented through a range of particular schemes that, by 1967, provided coverage for nearly the entire French population (Jambu-Merlin 1970, p. 12). This gradual extension made obsolete one of the principles of the 1851 Act on Public Hospitals, which stated that care in public hospitals would be open only to the indigent. The 1941 Act on Public Hospitals had already allowed physicians to treat private patients in paying beds of public hospitals. But the 1945 extension of health insurance benefits accelerated the influx of "nonindigent sick" into the public hospitals (Courquet 1971, p. 3). This evolution was confirmed in 1958 by Article L.679 of Regulation 58-1198, which states that public hospitals are to be open to anyone who is in need of care. Thereby, the growth of health insurance coverage contributed to the 1958 hospital reforms.

A second reason for the 1958 focus on hospitals resulted from the war. After World War II, France was confronted with the problem of a partly destroyed, partly obsolete, hospital infrastructure, with few resources available for reconstruction, renewal, or maintenance. The first national plan (covering 1947–1953) set priorities for postwar reconstruction that did not even touch on the health care sector. However, the second (1954–1957) and third (1958–1961) plans did recognize the development of hospitals as an important goal.

The differential development of public and private hospitals was a third reason for the 1958 reforms. Private hospitals, although eligible for social insurance reimbursement, were only under limited government regulations. So they saw fit to expand into profitable areas like surgery and obstetrics, leaving the more costly services (in terms of insurance coverage) like emergency services to the public hospitals.

A fourth reason for the 1958 hospital reforms was the gap between universities and teaching hospitals. The universities as research settings, and the hospitals as units of practical application, were not felt to be undertaking joint efforts or providing mutual enrichment. In 1956 a governmental committee led by Professor Debré was established to study this gap and some of the bottlenecks in the French health care system. The 1958 hospital reforms were based mainly on the results of this committee's work, and they are therefore sometimes called the Debré reforms. The reforms had three main goals (Comet 1965, p. 14):

1. to adapt hospital legislation to new technical developments
2. to prevent uncoordinated construction of public or private hospitals
3. to improve medical education and medical research

The 1958 Reforms in Review

An analysis of the 1958 hospital reforms and the legislation emanating from them could easily lead to the conclusion that the hospital is the most important element in the French health care system. Professor Pequignot warns, however, that such a conclusion underestimates the importance of nonhospital medicine. According to him, the discrepancy between the abundance of French hospital legislation and its real, rather limited, impact is due to the changes that took place in the French legislative process in 1958: since then, Parliament has only been able to put forward broad principles; the real power lies with the executive. Thus, the reaction of the executive determines whether the wishes of the legislature will be executed. According to Pequignot, the executive has, in this manner, blocked both the 1958 and the 1970 reforms. (Not every one of the French advisors we contacted for this study shares his opinion, however.) Whatever the case, the impression, at least, is very strong that the French national health care program is hospital-oriented.

The 1958 hospital reforms embodied a range of regulations, decrees, and other legislative instruments, of which three important sets of regulations represent its main objectives. First, Regulation 58-1198 on hospital legislation reform was intended to achieve three purposes (Ordonnance 58-1198):

1. to define the role of the public hospitals in the provision of health care
2. to assure the adequate functioning of the public hospitals—for example, by laying down requirements for the staffing of these hospitals
3. to set rules on the internal administration of public hospitals, which would be divided into four categories: regional hospital centers, hospital centers, hospitals, and rural hospitals

Regulation 58-1198 contained only general statements and referred to statutory regulations for more detail, specifically, to Decree 58-1202 on public hospitals (Décret 58-1202). The object of this decree was to achieve the second and third purposes of Regulation 58-1198.

1. To improve medical staffing of the public hospitals, the decree elaborated the principle of full-time service for physicians. It prescribed that regional hospital centers, and certain hospital centers designated by the minister, must appoint radiologists, pathologists, and anesthetists on a full-time basis. This principle has been called the most important innovation of the 1958 reforms.
2. For the internal administration of the public hospitals, the decree

provided a new composition for the administrative commission (board of trustees) by giving physicians, health insurance agencies, and other involved parties representation on this commission. Special provisions dealt with the representation of medical schools on teaching hospital boards. On the other hand, the decree also strengthened the authority of the hospital director. The introductory text to the decree stated that hospital management requires competence and knowledge that can only be achieved by professionals. Therefore, the decree (Article 26) required that the director and his staff have a specialized hospital management training at the National School of Public Health or in a health care institution (Décret 58-1202).

A second regulation, 58-1199, gave the minister of public health the responsibility for coordinating public and private hospitals (Ordonnance 58-1199). A procedure of preliminary declaration was introduced. No private hospital could be built or expanded without informing the minister. He could oppose the plans if they were not compatible with a number of technical requirements or, and this is important, if he considered the health care needs of the population already met by the existing facilities.

The third regulation, 58-1373 (Ordonnance 58-1373), on the creation of academic health sciences centers, contained two innovations:
1. Teaching hospitals and medical schools were merged. The regulation required each medical school to organize, in cooperation with the hospital center of the city in which it was located, the provision of health care, education, and research through an academic health sciences center. To this purpose both parties had to agree.
2. Dual-appointment status was established, which meant that the medical personnel of the hospital center would have to undertake teaching responsibilities, and university staff would have to carry clinical responsibilities.

Although the 1958 reforms were essentially directed at hospitals, they included important aspects of human resources development. In medical education, they tried to bridge the gap between teaching and research and between clinical practice and research. The principle of full-time medical staff in the leading hospitals was a fundamental change. The reforms also stressed hospital management professionalism, by reinforcing the responsibilities of the director and requiring him to be educated in an appropriate way.

1970: Hospital Reforms, a Second Round

After the 1958 reforms, the French hospital system was gradually confronted with an increasing competition between the public and private hospital sectors (Pruvost and Samson 1974). The private hospitals, having a flexible management, and not charged with a public mandate to cover all types of care, continued to thrive on lucrative specialties such as surgery and obstetrics. As a consequence, the public hospitals had to cope with growing financial difficulties (Inspection des affaires sociales 1972). The relationship between private and public hospitals became so strained and competitive that at one point the abolition of private hospitals was proposed (Blanpain 1975, p. 174).

This competition between the two hospital sectors had serious repercussions for the French health care system, since it led to wasteful and irrational distribution of services. The 1958 regulations on coordination of the two sectors seemed to have little effect, apart from stemming the expansion of the private sector. According to the explanatory note to the 1970 act, the two types of hospitals existed side by side without any functional interrelationship, unrelated to any overall plan, and subject to different sets of regulations. Moreover, the public hospitals were confronted with internal difficulties. The explanatory note to the 1970 act stated that the public hospitals suffered from isolation and an ambiguous legal status. The 1958 reforms had tried to classify them into four types, according to their size and the services they provided, but this classification did not include a functional hierarchy nor any schematic interrelationship. A public hospital's autonomy was considered to be excessive in certain circumstances and insufficient in others. Its governing body had no clearly defined power, and the medical staff were thought to have insufficient managerial responsibilities (Ministère de la Santé Publique 1970). Another problem that led to the 1970 reform was the widening gap between hospital-based physicians and community-based practitioners, general practitioners as well as specialists, who had no hospital privileges and thus could not keep abreast of and benefit from new technology, new diagnostic tools, and advanced treatment methods.

Keynotes of the 1970 Act (Loi du 31 décembre 1970)

Through a series of statutory regulations, the 1970 act aims at the implementation of two clear objectives: on the one hand, a cooperative and balanced relationship between the public and private hospitals; and, on the other, new interhospital structures and more flexible modes of hospital management (Ministère de la Santé Publique 1973). Probably the most important innovation of the 1970 act is the creation of a public hospital service. The public hospital service includes not only the public hospitals but also those private hospitals that wish to join it. The 1970 act offers three possibilities for private hospital participation. First, private nonprofit hospitals can join in a fully integrated way. In doing so they have the same rights and duties as public hospitals. Second, private profit hospitals can conclude a contract of concession with the state. In this contract, the state commits itself to refrain from approving the creation of any health care institution offering services similar to those of the contracting hospital. In principle this commitment is valid within certain time limits and in a given area. In return the hospital commits itself to take on the same duties as a public hospital. Finally, private hospitals can opt for an association agreement concerning specific services or patient groups.

The 1970 Act (Article 4) empowers the minister of public health to classify all hospitals, public as well as private, participating in the public hospital service. (The 1958 classification only applied to public hospitals.) The new act makes a distinction between acute general hospitals and extended-care institutions. A further division is based on the degree of advanced medical technology available in the hospital, permitting a vertical classification according to the level and variety of the health services that a hospital provides. In this way, the acute hospitals are divided into regional hospital centers, hospital centers, and local hospitals. To achieve a balanced supply of the different types of hospitals within the hospital service, the 1970 Act contains an authorization procedure for the creation and extension of private hospitals, based on a health facilities chart for France. This replaces the more arbitrary coordination procedure of the 1958 regulation.

The 1970 act also introduces new interhospital structures to remedy the lack of cooperation between hospitals. The two main new structures are the interhospital group and the interhospital syndicate. At the regional level, the regional hospital center, together with all the other institutions cooperating in the public hospital service, are legally required to form a regional interhospital group. The same institutions are entitled to form a regional interhospital syndicate. Interhospital groups have only consultative responsibilities and cannot act as corporations. Interhospital syndicates, on the other hand, can take on corporative responsibilities and can share services, train personnel, centralize services, and pool resources. According to Article 14 of the act, health care institutions that do not provide hospital treatment (such as general-practitioner group practices) can cooperate within the public hospital service through an interhospital group or an interhospital syndicate.

To make the management of public hospitals more dynamic and responsive, a new division of responsibilities between the board of trustees and the hospital director was introduced. The director benefited from this change in the balance of power. The responsibilities of the board were restricted, and the hospital director was empowered to execute the decisions of the board and to decide on all questions not specified in the act. The Federation of French Hospitals, representing the public hospitals, lobbied vigorously for this change in the responsibilities of the hospital administrator (Raynaud 1974, p. 12). Along the same line of promoting a more dynamic management, the act determines the conditions under which public hospitals can, in exceptional circumstances, borrow money to finance their investments.

A Balance of Power

The French Federation of Private Hospitals viewed the 1970 bill as an acceptable compromise between increased state intervention and continued liberty for private initiative. This balance of power had only been reached as a result of the federation's unyielding struggle against different government proposals threatening the very existence of private hospitals. The federation supported the 1970 bill because it signified the eventual recognition of the irreplaceable role of the private health care institutions. As to the actual content of the bill, the federation took a reserved position, since it seemed impossible to judge a bill that could only be implemented through a considerable number of statutory regulations. Only when these regulations had been published, they argued, could a definite viewpoint be determined. Furthermore, the federation noticed with regret that some attempts at "excessive" state intervention had not disappeared from the bill (Iba Zizen 1973, p. 169).

The Federation of French Hospitals, representing the public hospitals, welcomed the bill because it contained a number of elements favoring the influence and the development of the public hospitals. Discussion of the bill widened into a serious public debate on the different problems of the French hospital system. Through a number of articles, declarations, proposals, and comments, the Federation of French Hospitals was able to incorporate its viewpoints into the legislative process (Raynaud 1971). Hospital physicians mounted considerable opposition towards articles 27 and 28, empowering the hospital authorities to admit free-practicing physicians and midwives into the hospitals (Raynaud 1971, p. 15).

Human Resources

Medical manpower in France is generated by two streams of educational activities: on the one hand, the medical faculties of the universities; on the other, the teaching hospitals. Until 1971, entry into the system was unlimited, but progression through the different stages was controlled by rigorous examinations and by limited vacancies in internships, residencies, and house-staff positions in the teaching hospitals. Most of the students were in Paris, since the teaching capacity was concentrated there. Although curriculum content, examinations, and other matters were regulated by legislation, the actual number of doctors available was influenced more by student attrition. As Bridgman told us, the sums of money generated by the compulsory health insurance introduced in 1930 not only raised the standard of living for physicians but also, in his opinion, attracted more candidates to the study of medicine. Unfortunately, no data could be advanced to support this impression, although Sigerist was able to substantiate such a trend in Germany after the introduction of compulsory insurance there (Sigerist 1960). The issue of an eventual oversupply of physicians emerged in the late sixties. A surplus was envisioned and the act of July 12, 1971, introduced a selection procedure for admission to medical training. Training positions at second-year level were limited to 9,000, for which some 40,000 first-year students could compete (Le Monde, May 26, 1976). The health committee working on the seventh plan (1976–1980) projected that the density of 200 physicians per 100,000 inhabitants, established for 1985 in the sixth national plan, would almost be attained in 1980 (190 per 100,000), and the density would reach between 232 and 243 by 1985. As a result, a further reduction in the number of second-year positions open for competition was suggested; in May 1976 the state secretary for the universities announced that the government had in principle decided to reduce the 9,000 positions to 8,000 over the next five years, in ways still to be determined (*Le Monde,* May 26, 1976). At the same time, measures were announced to control the intake of students in pharmacy. In a position paper published in mid-1976, the French Confederation of Medical Unions strongly suggested that the number of second-year medical students be reduced even further, to 7,000 (Confédération des Syndicats Médicaux 1976).

The number of physicians is not the only problem in France. Indeed, regardless of the possibility of a rapid oversupply at current production rates, the uneven territorial distribution of physicians—more doctors in the north than in the south, more in urban areas than in rural areas—became worse between 1962 and 1972. (La Commission de la Santé 1976). On the average, the regional disparities vary from two-to-one for general practitioners to three-to-one for specialists. Some areas in Brittany have no physicians at all. Other underserved regions are Picardie, the Ardèche, and parts of Normandy. In January 1976 the Ministry of Health published a map showing the territorial distribution of medical resources, and indicating the gaps to be filled (Manévy 1976).

The health committee for the seventh plan is thus concerned with measures to correct the maldistribution of physicians and to affect the widespread tendency of medical graduates to begin practice in a location close to the academic health sciences centers where they were trained. But proposals to relocate academic health sciences centers, many of which are concentrated in and around Paris, are not considered feasible, nor are they welcomed by organized medicine. Therefore, the committee has suggested an increase in practice-training positions in underserved areas, to bring students there at the time when they are deciding where to locate (La Commission de la Santé 1976, p. 114). At the end of 1976, a special government committee, the Ordonneau Committee, was studying the conditions influencing the practice of medicine, with special attention to the problems of maldistribution (*Le Monde,* April 28, 1976b). French organized medicine is acutely aware of the difficulties created by physician maldistribution. Spokesmen for the French Confederation of Medical Unions have admitted that in the long run the right of free establishment of physicians cannot be maintained. Meanwhile, special incentives are suggested to redirect distribution. However, opinions about the nature of these incentives vary. Some favor special loans at low interest rates for doctors prepared to go to underserved areas. Others prefer fiscal exemptions. Still others stress the creation of group practice centers, on the assumption that the prospect of mutual help is an important factor in a physician's decision to work in underserved areas, where the spectre of overwork and isolation is a discouraging factor. Development of rural hospitals and salaried medical posts in town halls of rural regions are also suggested.

Another dimension in the debate on physician supply and physician distribution is the implementation of provisions of the Treaty of Rome, which determines the relations of the member countries of the European Economic Community. As of December 16, 1976, a physician who is a national of one of the nine Common Market countries can, when he meets the mutual recognition (minimal) requirements, establish practice in any other country of the European Community (Blanpain 1975, p. 267–78). Nearly 20 years of difficult negotiations preceded this first step in the making of the "white" Europe, a term coined as a complement to the so-called "green" Europe—the common market for agriculture. French representatives in these negotiations for a long time took issue with the application of the Treaty of Rome to doctors employed in public hospitals. They claimed that foreign physicians could not qualify for positions in public hospitals because the treaty excludes employment in public service from the free movement of labor, which was the provision on which the free circulation of physicians was to be based. Representatives of the other countries argued that physicians in public hospitals cannot be considered as public employees in the true legal sense because of their clinical autonomy (Blanpain 1973). Eventually, the member-countries were encouraged to make medical positions in public hospitals accessible to nationals of other member-countries.

Employment of physicians in public hospitals has been an ongoing issue in France for other reasons. The establishment of full-time status for physicians was an important objective of the 1958 hospital reforms. Mechanisms were introduced to increase full-time medical staff, including: two salaries for those having dual appointments to a hospital and a university, a fee-pool resulting from private outpatients and inpatients seen under defined conditions on the hospital premises, and more rapid advancement opportunities in the career structure. These mechanisms were introduced first in the teaching hospitals and later in the regional hospitals. With the tendency of the French legislative process to go into very detailed regulation, this movement towards full-time hospital staff involved a lot of controversy over fundamentally trivial issues in the implementation phase and generated many articles and letters to the editors in the medical journals at the time.

While studying the issue of full-time hospital staff in February 1961, at the French Ministry of Health, Jan Blanpain was told that part of the tendency to go into extreme regulatory detail was due to the unusually high ratio of female to male civil servants at the Ministry of Health! Under the Vichy government during World War II, a number of vacancies in the career ladder were filled by an unusually rapid progression of hard-working female civil servants. The strong presence of this group, it was said, had resulted in a different style of executive attention, with an emphasis on minutiae and detail. Needless to say, the spokesman was male.

Eventually the movement for full-time medical staff in hospitals got under way. By 1965, 40 percent of the medical staff of regional hospital centers and academic health sciences centers was on a full-time basis, and in 1972 this figure had risen to 81 percent. The percentage was higher in the university hospitals than in the regional centers (Ministère de la Santé Publique 1973, p. 71). Vacancies continue to exist in public hospitals (Raynaud 1974), however, particularly in fields like gynecology, radiology, and biology: in June 1975, there were 388 listed vacancies for full-time department heads in general hospitals (La Commission de la Santé, p. 143). This type of shortage, combined with an oversupply of physicians and the limits on the free establishment of individual practice, have directed more and more medical graduates into specialization. The declining percentage of general practitioners, down to 62 percent of the medical manpower in 1969, although still high compared to other countries (35 percent in the United States in 1969), reflects the functional maldistribution to which new manpower initiatives sought to respond (Rösch 1973, p. 141). A revision of general practitioner education is considered necessary (Le Monde, April 28, 1976a). The Fougère

Committee has proposed to add a special module for general practitioner education to the normal medical curriculum (*Le Monde,* March 17, 1976). During their March 1976 assembly at Nancy, the deans of French medical schools discussed a similar approach (*Le Monde,* May 26, 1976). Meanwhile, in the broader European context, a harmonization of general practitioner training is being pursued in conjunction with the agreed requirements for mutual recognition of diplomas.

The supply of allied health professionals has been a predominantly hospital-based responsibility. Enormous efforts were made in France during the sixties to increase the quantity of nonmedical personnel, especially in the public hospitals. Since 1968 their number has grown at a rate of 7.5 percent per year, although this increase is still considered too small to meet the needs. These inadequacies are due partly to a significant rate of attrition during the first years of employment (because of low status and remuneration) and partly to the small capacity of the schools (Sénat 1973, p. 571).

In the nursing schools, however, this capacity has grown considerably: in 1974 each department had at least one nursing school, and the number of first-year students increased from 13,000 in 1969 to 22,000 in 1975–76. This increase has been accompanied by a growing supply of nurses: 270 per 100,000 in 1969 against 349 per 100,000 in 1974. The public hospitals employed 45,000 nurses in 1969, 68,700 in 1974. These improvements have been achieved through deliberate actions to ameliorate both the circumstances of the students (studies are completely free) and subsequent employment conditions (career structure and growing remuneration). However, the health committee for the seventh plan estimates the current shortage of nursing personnel in public hospitals at 20 percent, a shortage that is even more pronounced in Paris, Bourgogne, and the North. The committee proposes a twofold policy to tackle the problem: improve the working conditions in public hospitals, and increase the intake capacity of the nursing schools to 25,000 a year (La Commission de la Santé 1976, p. 145).

The development of health administrators has been focused mainly on the needs of hospital management. In 1945, a National School of Public Health was created in Paris and was then transferred to excellent new facilities built for it on the new campus of Rennes University in 1963. This school is responsible for undergraduate and graduate training in hospital administration, as well as education in public health practice, environmental hygiene, epidemiology, and health education. The training schemes relate to career paths of civil servants selected on the basis of national examinations (World Health Organization 1972, p. 9). The 1958 and 1970 hospital reforms provided momentum for the professional education of hospital managers, by increasing the hospital manager's responsibilities and by making formal qualifications for a hospital administrative position mandatory. The move of the National School of Public Health to Rennes was part of a general policy of regional development and decentralization from Paris. A number of people have since questioned the wisdom of this transfer; the distance, requiring several hours of travel, makes communication between the hub of health policy decision-making and a potential think-tank (the only French school of public health) difficult.

The development of health consumerism has been very limited in France. The many sickness funds in operation before the introduction of compulsory health insurance in 1930 have been greatly reduced in number. The supervision of health care, like most other government functions in France, remains strongly centralized and administered from Paris. The medical profession in France has maintained its traditional powerful status vis-à-vis the government and the sickness funds. In this context, it is not surprising that there is no officially supported consumer voice in French medical affairs; so far, even the idea has appeared unthinkable to most health professions. For example, a note from the Federation of French Hospitals, on November 21, 1972, on the topic "the right of intervention in the hospital by consumers," rejected out of hand a number of different possibilities of consumer involvement.

A partial justification for this position is that in France there is a strong paternalistic attitude towards the patient. In a 1971 report on health care policies, delivered to the then minister of public health and social security, M. Robert Boulin, seventy-seven pages were devoted to "humanizing the hospital." Minute directions are given on how the patient should be admitted to the hospital, the physical environment of the ward, and the human atmosphere with which the patient should be surrounded, consistent with the attention for detail. How the patient could secure his rights to these conditions or how his grievances might be received is not discussed; but the general thrust is that health personnel should be nice to the patient and remember that he is a sick human being. The regulations specified are laudatory, and do not exist in such detail in other European countries.

There are two large and well-organized consumer organizations in France, the Institut National de Consommation, and the Union Fédérale des Consommateurs. They have studied subjects such as nutrition, food purity, and the safety of toys, but neither has undertaken studies in medical care as such. No patients' associations or pressure groups, other than the familiar organizations like the Heart Association, have been identified.

Physical Resources

Hospitals

The first French hospital was established privately in the sixth century by a religious order. During the French Revolution, in 1794, all French hospitals were nationalized. However, this nationalization was a financial catastrophe. Two years later, in 1796, under the Directoire, the hospitals were transferred to the municipalities; among these hospitals, the private hospitals were given back to the religious orders. Then, during the nineteenth century, private profit-making hospitals began to be established (Aujaleu, p. 120). With the exception of an act of 1838 that required each department to have a psychiatric hospital, the first government intervention in the development of health care institutions after the French Revolution was the 1941 Act on Public Hospitals. This act was important because it made the public hospitals accessible to everyone, and removed them from the "care of the indigent" sphere. The act also increased the central government's control over public hospitals by allocating new responsibilities for the opening and maintaining of public general hospitals, especially to the departmental prefects, and by establishing a committee to evaluate the utilization and financial resources of every French public hospital.

A second, more important step, was taken in 1954. Before then, state support for building hospitals had been limited and irregular. New technological developments, the use of very expensive and rapidly obsolete equipment, and the recognition of the right to health care now required the government to intervene—at least financially—in a more regular and substantial way. At the same time, the government decided to integrate such efforts in the four-year plans

(Ministère de la Santé Publique 1973, p. 49). The first of these national development plans, covering the period 1947–1953, had not even mentioned health care facilities: immediately after World War II all available resources had to be used for the reconstruction of major industries such as steel, chemistry, and transport, and nothing was left for hospital renewal. But the second plan (1954–1957) recognized the need to develop health care facilities. This recognition was based upon a departmental and regional survey of the existing hospitals, conducted from 1944 onwards in preparation for the second plan, and also upon studies of the hospital needs of the population. These studies revealed an inadequate situation, quantitatively and qualitatively. The second plan therefore proposed that 300 million francs be invested in health care and social care facilities, instead of the annual 6 million francs. Out of a list of 600 proposed projects, 180 were selected as national priorities, and became eligible for a 40 percent state subsidy of the investment costs.

The health aspects of the second plan had been prepared at the local level by the prefects and at the national level by the Ministry of Health and the General Planning Office, assisted by a Health and Social Services Facilities Committee. The second plan did not, however, result in comprehensive hospital planning, because it dealt with public hospitals and nonprofit private institutions only. It left the private profit institutions completely alone. Although bound to respect certain technical requirements, these last hospitals were not otherwise supervised or controlled (Aujaleu, p. 121). Thus, they functioned in virtually complete freedom, while at the same time subscribers to social insurance and their dependents were free to choose to be treated in them, with their hospitalization costs refunded on the same basis as in public or private nonprofit institutions. This situation contributed to the 1958 hospital reforms and to the introduction of the obligation for private hospitals to notify the ministry of their building intentions. Although its basic objective was to provide some coordination between public and private initiative, the coordination measure introduced in 1958 resulted mainly in a number of ministerial refusals to acknowledge the need for building or adding of new private beds: between 1959 and 1970 the percentage of applications for bed-extensions that were approved dropped from 60 percent to 33 percent (Ministère de la Santé Publique 1973, p. 110). Meanwhile, the construction of public hospitals, begun following the second plan, continued during the period of the third plan (1958–1961), although fewer were built in 1958 and 1959, because of the weak economic situation at that time (Ministère de la Santé Publique 1973, p. 50).

Despite this effort, by 1954 the need for more balanced hospital planning had been recognized, and Regulation 58-1199 (Ordonnance 58-1199) and Decree 58-1202 (Décret 58-1202) established a National Committee for Hospital Care, responsible for preparing an inventory of the population's health care needs and the corresponding supply of public hospital beds, and further for advising on the construction, conversion, or closure of public hospitals. The committee had also to advise on the National Development and Equipment Plan and on its priorities.

During the early sixties France experienced a clear trend towards regionalization and sectorization. This trend was important in the development of health services planning, because the idea of a hospital facilities chart and a health facilities chart eventually emerged from it (Ministère de la Santé Publique 1973, p. 126). The implementation of regionalization began with a circular of March 15, 1960, which divided up the departments into psychiatric sectors. Another important step towards regionalization was the preparation of the fifth plan (1966–1970). The circular of May 28, 1963, on the preparation of this plan, contained a number of directives calling for regionalization. The detailed preparation of the fifth plan was itself done by region, and the procedure for preparing the plan was changed. The earlier plans had been detailed at both the local and national level; since the preparation of the fifth plan, regional prefects have played an important role in the planning of health care facilities in each region (Ecole Nationale de la Santé 1974, p. 28).

Especially during 1969 and 1970, the executive issued several circulars propounding the idea of regionalization and sectorization. The most important of these circulars was that of December 26, 1969, on the preparation of the sixth plan. The main purpose of this circular was to stimulate a study of the need for hospital beds. The country was divided into a large number of health care sectors, grouped into twenty-one larger health care regions. These regions have played an important role in establishing the health facilities chart that presents the boundaries of health care sectors and in preparing an inventory of existing facilities and of those required in the near future (Ministère de la Santé Publique 1974, p. 128). The idea of establishing health care sectors, health care regions, and a health facilities chart was embodied legally in the 1970 Hospital Reform Act. This health facilities chart can be reviewed at any time, and it has to be reviewed compulsorily each time a new national development and equipment plan is being prepared. The health facilities chart is prepared by the minister of public health, together with the minister of social affairs, upon consultation with regional committees and a national committee. These committees are composed of representatives of the ministries involved, the local authorities, the sickness funds, and the private and public hospitals.

According to Article 47 of the 1970 act, the health facilities chart has a twofold function: first, it serves as the basis for planning and programming of all health care facilities—private as well as public— that participate in the public hospital service; second, it provides the elements for the "authorization" procedure, introduced in 1967 to replace the 1958 requirement of declaration of building intentions. This means that no health care institution—private or public—can be built in France if it does not fit into the health facilities chart (Ministère de la Santé Publique 1973, p. 130). The procedure introduced in 1958 was transformed by Decree 67-829 of September 23, 1967. Following this decree, the preliminary declaration was replaced by a preliminary authorization to be awarded by the minister of public health. The 1970 act confirmed this 1967 decree, although with some modifications: the extension of the certification-of-need procedure to expensive technology; the toughening of the criteria for authorization; and the regionalization of the decision-making process. The authorization is given by the regional prefect, after advice from a regional hospital committee. The decision of the prefect can be appealed by any interested party; the minister of public health has to decide on such appeals within six months, after seeking the advice of a national committee. The regional committees and the national committee are presided over by a magistrate, and are composed of representatives of the medical unions, the Ministry of Public Health, the sickness funds, the hospitals cooperating in the public hospital service, and the private hospitals. Six years after the publication of the 1970 act, the cooperation among private and public hospitals in the public hospital service is negligible. The commission on the seventh plan has recommended that the statutory regulations required to implement the act be established as soon as possible (La Commission de la Santé 1976, p. 133).

Social security agencies have always been very important in the development of hospitals in France. The regulations of October 1945 enabled the social insurance funds to create a special development fund with a national center and regional branches. This fund receives a percentage of the total budget of each main social insurance branch, determined each year by a ministerial regulation (Bridgman 1971, p. 388). However, social insurance organizations cannot decide freely to establish or to subsidize any health institution. Their proposals must fit within the health facilities chart. Moreover, the regional branches of the special fund, presided over by the prefect, decide on the distribution of the subsidies, grants, or loans. There is, therefore, no risk that the social insurance funds will support institutions outside the national plan. At present, the health insurance agencies play a twofold function in the development of French hospitals, serving both as administrators and as financing agencies. They are involved in administration in three ways. First, they administer the hospitals they have established. According to some sources, the health insurance agencies intend to increase the building of their own hospitals (Inspection générale des affaires sociales 1972). Second, the health insurance agencies participate in the administration of the public hospitals. Finally, the agencies are represented on the regional and national hospital committees and on the regional and national committees charged with preparing the health services chart.

As financing agencies, the health insurance agencies finance the hospitals they construct. In refunding the per diem costs for hospitals, they make allowance for the costs of capital depreciation. Furthermore, the agencies operate as important health care investment bankers. The classic scheme by which public hospitals in France are financed involves 40 percent from state subsidies, 30 percent from loans from health insurance agencies, and 30 percent from loans in the usual capital market (Mandeville 1974, p. 238). Therefore, the health insurance agencies in France have been called by one author the permanent investment bank of the French hospital system (Polack 1971, p. 164).

Health Centers

The health insurance agencies have also played a significant role in the development of health centers and group practices in France. Immediately after World War II, the health insurance agencies proposed that French physicians should practice as employees of a company financed entirely or to a great extent by the social security institutions. But the Confederation of French Medical Unions rejected the proposal. Another proposal recommended the formation of two associations for each health center, one of which would own the health center and the other comprising the physicians who would practice in the center, renting the facility from the first association. This proposal also failed.

Since then, physicians have found ways to raise financial support for the establishment of health centers and group practices on their own. As an example, there is a mutual fund supported by the Pension Fund of French Physicians. This resulted from an agreement between the pension fund and the Confederation of French Medical Unions to use the fund's assets for loans at low interest rates to physicians, for the construction of health centers, and so on. The mutual fund has contributed considerbly to the success of medical centers in France. Moreover, the Confederation of French Medical Unions and the National Association of Physicians in Group Practice have been pressuring important banks to lend money to their members for the construction of such centers (Guiheneuf 1967).

Information Resources

Health Research

Although the French national government has traditionally had a strong hand in organizing and coordinating all sectors of public life, until recently health research in France has been fairly disorganized. Until 1940, nearly all health research was undertaken either in independent university faculties or in the Pasteur Institute, a private foundation that supported research out of its income from vaccines, sera, and the manufacture of laboratory products. Although even before the war the government wanted to organize research, it was not until about 1960 that some coherence was achieved. There were two reasons for the delay. First, World War II drastically upset all research activity and many research teams were disbanded; four years of isolation put French biomedical research back in comparison with the Anglo-Saxon countries. Second, immediately after the war, in an effort to speed up reconstruction and development, the French government gave absolute priority to research in physics, chemistry, and mathematics, and curtailed development of biomedical and health services research. In the sixties, some coordination was finally achieved, and a pattern was established that has determined health research policy and activity in France until the present day. This pattern of coordination emerged from the successive creation of research institutions, each of which derived from the preceding institution and stimulated the following one.

(1) The Delegation for Scientific and Technical Research (Blanpain and Delesie 1976, p. 146), created in 1958 and organized in 1961, was attached to the prime minister's office until 1970. It was then attached to the minister of industrial and scientific development, although it still retains considerable independence and is actually responsible to an Interministerial Committee on Scientific and Technical Research, a high-powered research policy body. The delegation's authority for establishing research policy, including health research, is the greatest in France. It prepares national plans for economic and social development on matters of research and development. Hence, it actually sets priorities. It centralizes the budgets of all research proposals submitted to government agencies, and follows them up through research budget control. It has its own funds available for any specific priority research it wishes: such projects are referred to as "concerted actions." Finally, it is strongly represented on the boards of specialized research institutes such as INSERM. The delegation has been empowered to determine and implement directly or indirectly any research policy in France. In this task, it succeeds pretty well. Specific priority areas designated by the delegation are nearly all oriented towards biomedical research: for example, molecular actions in biology, biological and medical engineering, immunology or organ transplants (Burg 1973, p. 69).

(2) The National Institute of Public Health and Medical Research (INSERM). The decline of the university-oriented National Center for Scientific Research, which traditionally held the most power in the field of scientific research, led to the creation of INSERM by the minister of health. By the sixties the National Center had proven unable to cope with changing needs. While the Delegation for Scientific and Technical Research is oriented primarily toward health research policy, INSERM is oriented toward research activity. The bulk of medical research in France is either undertaken or financed by INSERM. About half of INSERM research is intramural, while the

other half is undertaken by research groups in other laboratories under direct contract. With the growing emphasis on health research during the sixties, INSERM's funds increased. In 1973, some 125 intramural research units, with an average of eight researchers per unit, were in operation. INSERM has a specific division of health services research, consisting of eleven sections, of which the most important are the section on statistics, epidemiology, and information services; the section on mortality and morbidity statistics; and the section on public health strategies.

(3) The Medical Economy Division of the Center for Research and Documentation of Consumption (CREDOC). Just as the minister of health created INSERM in the early sixties to launch his own research efforts, the General Planning Office attached to the prime minister's office had even earlier created CREDOC, in 1954, to support its own research activities. Since the mid-sixties, and as a result of the renewed emphasis on health and medical research in France, CREDOC has flourished. It consists of six divisions that provide the necessary research and statistical back-up for the development of national plans for socioeconomic development. The division on medical economy is particularly important with respect to health. Although its statistical objective is certainly the most important, its research activities within the area of health services are especially significant in the development of health delivery priorities. These research activities include macroeconomic analysis of health accounts, macroeconomic analysis of the health care system, surveys of medical care consumption, and miscellaneous studies, such as work patterns of general practitioners.

(4) The National Center for Scientific Research (Blanpain and Delesie 1976, p. 149), founded in 1939 within the Ministry of Education, was the traditional stronghold of university-based research. The National Center's research strategy was based upon a single-discipline approach and administration by decision-making bodies with a rigid membership. Essentially, this strategy resulted in its own decline. Although the center tried to counteract this decline, for instance, by introducing programmed cooperative research efforts in 1959, such efforts were not a success. Only in 1970, when the Delegation for Scientific and Technical Research, INSERM, and CREDOC were already well established in health research, was the center able to develop a coherent research policy, based upon a thorough reorganization of the universities after the May revolt of 1968. This

renewed research policy was implemented through "programmed thematic actions" and a reorganization of the center's budget so that the center's directors have funds to allocate at their own discretion.

(5) The Pasteur Institute, originally a private foundation, began to receive important government grants in 1968. Many Pasteur Institute researchers are also supported by the National Center or by IN-SERM. The Institute is particularly active in the areas of molecular biology, immunology, and microbiology (Blanpain and Delesie 1976, p. 156).

(6) The Section on PPBS and Operations Research of the Office of Research and Planning. Although by 1970 a number of institutions had already taken initiatives in health research, each within its own area, it was nevertheless felt that in a country such as France, where centralized socioeconomic policy and development were at least formally accorded much attention, coordination was a structural necessity. The creation of a Ministry of Industrial and Technical Development in 1969, the reorganization of higher education at the same period, and the merger of the Ministry of Health and the Ministry of Social Security in 1970 all reflect this effort to bring about coordination at the highest level. Within the renewed Ministry of Health and Social Affairs, this development was matched by the creation of the Bureau of Studies and Budgets, and its Section on PPBS and Operations Research. The section's objective is to provide scientific back-up for the Ministry's policy on health and social security. Its main methodology is to develop models by which the impact of any action upon the health system—its organization and its financing on the one hand, and its resources on the other hand—can be determined. Although only recently begun, the section's work looks promising.

The history and development of these six major health research institutions in France may create the impression that one is dealing with an explicit long-term research policy developed by the Central Planning Office attached to the Prime Minister's Office and implemented through the mechanism of the recurrent national plans. However, this does not in fact seem to be the case. The national plans are rather a historical record of political decisions taken in an interministerial committee, proposed and defended by the respective ministers in response to mid-term problems and in view of mid-term political feasibility. In a moment of exaggeration, it has even been suggested that the minister of finance wields more power over health and health research policy than the minister of education or the minister of health. Realistically, the health research trend may reflect a streamlining effort by the ministries of education and health to effect financial freedom of action, rather than a long-term policy that happens to have certain financial implications. Only since 1960 has health been included as an important aspect of national economic and social development. The fifth national plan (1966–1970) underlined the need for fundamental or basic research. The sixth plan (1971–1975) stressed the need for mission-oriented and implementation-oriented research.

Health Statistics

The development of health information systems often runs hand in hand with the development of health research. While particular data banks may reveal problem areas for further research, specific research efforts stress equally often the need for the development of usable information systems. Some differences in emphasis may, nevertheless, be discernible in individual countries. In France as a general rule (in contrast, for example, to the Netherlands), the development of an information system follows specific research results.

The National Institute for Statistics and Economic Studies, which is more a ministry division than an independent institution, was founded in 1946 to collect and keep current all statistics relevant to the country's socioeconomic life; it is also responsible for the national accounts. As might be expected, the institute's activities quickly became relevant to the activities of the prime minister's Central Planning Office and its national plans. The institute did not actually become specifically involved in detailed health information systems until health became part of the plans around the mid-fifties. Meanwhile the institute concentrated on such basic statistics as physical goods, their availability, production and consumption, both in value and volume.

When CREDOC was created in 1954, it was stipulated that half of CREDOC's board should be nominated by the minister of economy and finance. Because of this deliberate link with the National Institute for Statistics and Economic Studies, together with day-to-day contacts with a rather active group of researchers and administrators, by 1960 CREDOC had actually established itself as the statistical and research bureau for health care consumption statistics both in prices and in volume. CREDOC basically has three information systems. (1) Macro-economic analysis of health accounts: CREDOC developed the methodology and implemented very detailed health accounts and accounting-oriented data files, which are actually being promoted as models for the member countries of the European Economic Community. (2) Macro-economic analysis of the health care system: this implies a thorough analysis and development of supply and demand variables and files with respect to health care. (3) Medical care consumption analysis, for which CREDOC conducts extensive surveys (10,000 families—600 communities) on a regular basis—every ten years so far—to determine consumption patterns and to investigate shifts in relation to economic and social variables, epidemiological variables, and supply variables.

Four agencies within or attached to the Ministry of Health and Social Affairs are charged with the development of health information systems:

(1) The Office of Research and Statistics within the Bureau of Studies and Budgets keeps track of ordinary statistics—such as number of beds by public or private sector, by specialty, by region and so on—and some elementary utilization rates—such as number of admissions and lengths of stay. The Section of PPBS and Operations Research of the Office of Research and Planning within the same bureau has recently been trying to improve the ministry's statistical capability. Although the section is primarily research-oriented, it is well aware of current data shortcomings and, subject to the usual administrative constraints, is trying to do something about the problem. The lack of a national hospital institute in France precludes an information system for hospital activity like those of surrounding countries. For instance, no statistics are available on manpower or on diagnosis incidence rates within hospitals.

(2) The National Health Insurance Agency maintains traditional accounts statistics, such as number of physician services, following the nomenclature defined by a legal act, by health insurance agency conscription, and group of subscribers. The development of an information system based upon the National Health Insurance Agency data bank is now being undertaken by CREDOC.

(3) The National School of Public Health is active primarily in the area of health information systems methodology. As such, its statis-

tics section has initiated a four-year project to develop and implement an automated record system for handicapped persons and their health care needs.

(4) The National Institute of Public Health and Medical Research (INSERM) was founded with the objectives not only of undertaking biomedical research, but also of keeping the minister up to date on the country's health status. However, there is an imbalance between these two objectives, since only 10 percent of the institute's budget goes to the Health Services Research Division, which is charged with the second objective. This situation is due to historical circumstances: a research backlog, which resulted from a long period of inactivity between 1945 and 1960, and the decision-making structure of the institute, which favors medical and biomedical professionals. While the development of vital and health statistics and their information systems (very much comparable to the National Center for Health Statistics in the United States) preoccupies the Health Services Research Division, promising work has started recently to develop specific, application-oriented public health programs and health information systems. Examples are: the identification of health care problems of migrant workers in urban areas; the development, implementation, and management of an automated vaccination record file; and the development of an automated information system for preventive care, which started in 1971 and was tested with respect to tuberculosis in one of the French provinces. In close cooperation with the Section of PPBS and Operations Research of the Ministry of Public Health and Social Affairs, the division also tries to remedy the current lack of specific hospital utilization and hospital patient information systems. A nearly total lack of hospital activity data and hospital patient statistics precludes the prediction of the impact of particular hospital policy actions. Nevertheless, an optimal national hospital and health care plan is now envisioned and even required by law in France. As a result the Section of PPBS and Operations Research of the Office of Research and Planning of the Ministry of Health and Social Affairs is now launching a major effort to gather the data and analyze the statistics necessary, with a view to implementing a systems approach, which was required by the 1970 Hospital Act. The fact that even in 1975 very little of this health systems approach had been realized, not even in a pilot situation, is not at all surprising, given the enormous efforts required and the inertia to be overcome.

In Retrospect

The main thrust for the national health program in France has been provided by the social security system and its gradual extension over the years to cover the entire population. It created the money streams that supported resource development and it accommodated to a medical profession jealously guarding its prerogatives. Great efforts have been devoted to lifting the French public hospital system from a history of indigent care into a central role for modern health care and to bringing public and private initiatives into an alliance for the people's health.

5 | The Netherlands

Within a tradition of voluntary insurance, the Dutch had been considering compulsory health insurance for four decades when the German occupation forces abruptly forced their hand and introduced national health insurance in 1941 (Ziekenfondsenbesluit 1941). A second important episode in the Dutch national health program was the introduction of catastrophic illness insurance in 1967, the so-called Exceptional Medical Expenses Act (Wet 14 december 1967). From then on, the Netherlands moved only gradually towards greater control over its health care system. In 1974 an important policy proposal was introduced in Parliament to structure and rationalize the health care system and to contain health care costs (Ministerie van Volksgezondheid 1974). This proposal, which has recently resulted in major bills on health resources provision and on the restriction of health care prices, is the third episode selected for analysis in this study.

Preparing for Compulsory Health Insurance (1904–1941) and the 1941 Sickness Funds Decree

Several attempts to introduce compulsory health insurance were made in the Netherlands from 1904 on. In that year the Kuyper government introduced a bill providing cash benefits as well as benefits in kind, obviously based on the Bismarck legislation of 1883 in Germany. However, Dutch physicians were great adversaries of the Kuyper bill and of the similar bill presented by Kuyper's successor, Veegens, in 1907. They objected to the combination of cash benefits and benefits in kind (direct provision of care) and to the administration of both by the sickness funds. The doctors feared that employers and employees would dominate these funds as they had managed to do in Germany. Indeed, as stipulated in both bills, employers and employees would have each paid a part of the premium, which would have reduced enormously the influence of the physicians on the sickness funds. Another point of criticism concerned the ceiling of 1,200 florins below which all wage earners would be compulsorily insured. The physicians considered this ceiling too high, because they feared that it would reduce their income from private middle-class patients (Huysmans 1973, p. 139). Thus, neither of these bills were enacted.

A few years later, Minister Talma accommodated the physicians by introducing a new bill providing only cash benefits. Talma argued that benefits in kind should be regulated separately, because cash benefits are a response to the constant threat that illness poses to the income of wage earners, whereas benefits in kind (health care) meet the needs of non-wage-earners as well (Ministerie van Sociale Zaken 1966, p. 22). Talma's bill maintained a subtle link between cash benefits and benefits in kind, however, in the sense that only those who could prove their voluntary membership in a sickness fund (which entitled them to benefits in kind) were entitled to cash benefits: as such, this bill contained an indirect obligation to be insured for benefits in kind, and it laid down requirements for those sickness funds that wished to be involved in the administration of the benefits in kind (Van Langendonck 1971, p. 119).

Enacted in 1913, it was not until 1930 that Talma's Sickness Act came into force, at which time all the articles regarding the sickness funds had been eliminated. Furthermore, no regulations were issued regarding the indirect obligation to join a voluntary sickness fund in order to be eligible for cash benefits. This situation was to last until 1941. The stalling on such an important issue was due to the proposal made by Aalberse in 1920, a new bill containing a government-subsidized voluntary insurance scheme, which itself had little chance of success given the unfortunate economic circumstances of the period (Festen 1974, p. 367).

Nongovernmental groups also tried to regulate the sickness funds. The most outstanding initiative was taken just after the failure of the Aalberse bill in 1922 by the Dutch Organization of Labor Unions. A commission was formed with representatives from the unions, from the sickness funds controlled by the insured, and from doctors', dentists', and pharmacists' associations. This commission tried to unify the sickness funds. The commission was known as the Unification Commission and brought out the Unification Report. Although the report was not accepted by the membership of the represented organizations (the Roman Catholic Union began to establish its own sickness funds), it deeply influenced the development of the Dutch health insurance (Ledeboer 1966, p. 5).

In the 1930s the world-wide economic crisis was the main obstacle to a sickness funds act. In the Second Chamber of Parliament, Minister Verschuur declared that such an act would be too luxurious (Huysmans 1973, p. 169). The last attempt before World War II came from Minister Slingerberg who in 1936 proposed a fourth amendment to the Aalberse bill of 1920. A few years later it was cancelled by his successor, Minister Romme (Festen 1974, p. 383). The Netherlands entered the war in 1940 in the following situation: cash benefits had been provided since 1930 by the Talma Act, while the provision of benefits in kind was not regulated at all and remained on a voluntary basis. Almost one-half of the Dutch population was voluntarily insured with one of the 650 sickness funds. The funds all operated locally, and the income ceiling above which no one could be admitted was not uniform: traditionally, it was lower in the funds controlled by the Medical Association and by physicians (Ledeboer 1966, p. 5). Financing was provided through contributions from employers and employees, mostly lump sums independent of income. Government grants did not exist. The amount of contributions required differed for each fund, and as a result benefits also varied. In general these benefits consisted of medical care from general practitioners; obstetric care from a midwife or a general practitioner, or a lump sum in case of birth; drugs; specialist medical care to a limited extent; and, in towns, dental care, also to a limited and varying degree. Since the funds did not cover inpatient care, there also existed so-called hospital care associations, especially in the rural areas, but their coverage of hospital costs was very limited. Only the payment of the general practitioners, based on a capitation fee, showed a certain uniformity. Providers of care were in principle paid directly by the funds, without any financial intervention by the insured himself (although in some cases, for example, dental care benefits, copayment was required). Payment was based on agreements between local funds and individual providers; thus there existed widely different arrangements for the same type of provider.

Gradually, agreements became more standardized, as a result of collective bargaining between the professional organizations of providers and groups of funds (Internationale Vereniging voor Sociale Zekerheid 1959, p. 24).

Around the time when the Netherlands were invaded by the German armies (May 10, 1940), the minister of social affairs, van den Tempel, introduced a new bill on the sickness funds. This bill contained only general rules concerning the internal structure and administration of the funds, and established an indirect compulsory health insurance (providing benefits in kind), based on the Talma Sickness Act of 1913; this meant that the relevant article of the 1913 Sickness Act would finally come into force. The different parties (sickness funds, unions, the Medical Association, and so on), seeing that the Germans had their own plans for the sickness funds, displayed an unprecedented unity in accepting the van den Tempel Bill. According to the Germans, however, any health insurance scheme had to include two main provisions: first, a combination of cash benefits and benefits in kind directly compulsory for all wage earners, without any income ceiling; and second, financing through contributions, of which one-half was payable by the employer, the other by the employee. On these two important points, the bill clashed with the German ideas. Regardless of these conflicting views, the General Kommissar für Finanz und Wirtschaft, Jacob, introduced a German scheme, which had the following characteristics:

It was directly compulsory.
It offered benefits in kind as well as cash benefits.
The benefits in kind were administered by one state sickness fund, while the cash benefits were administered by the prevailing occupational organizations.
It was financed through contributions.

The sickness funds, the physicians, and the Medical Association were firmly against this plan. The Germans finally compromised and implemented the van den Tempel Bill in a very simplified and amended form as the Sickness Funds Decree of 1941.

Why did the Germans show such haste in introducing sickness insurance? Basically, there were two reasons. First, they were interested in the sickness funds for political and propaganda reasons; through social improvements they hoped to gain sympathy for National Socialism. Second, by forcing the Dutch employers to contribute to the financing of social insurance, they hoped to harmonize the competing position of German and Dutch industry, since German employers were already contributing to the costs of German health insurance (Mannoury 1966).

Scope and Content of the 1941 Decree

This decree introduced two new characteristics (Ziekenfondsraad 1965, p. 2): compulsory insurance for all wage earners having an income below the ceiling stipulated in the Sickness Act of 1913 and supervision of the sickness funds. The compulsory insurance provision meant that employers and employees were compelled to pay a contribution toward benefits in kind and that sickness funds were obliged to accept every wage earner having an income below the Sickness Act ceiling. But the decree itself did not contain an article compelling those earning wages below the ceiling to join a sickness fund. Membership in a sickness fund was, however, the exclusive way to be entitled to benefits in kind, as well as the only way to enjoy cash benefits, since Talma's 1913 Sickness Act had made the receipt of cash benefits dependent on sickness fund membership. Outside this compulsory scheme, sickness funds continued to operate on a voluntary basis for insured with incomes above the ceiling set in the 1913 Sickness Act. The ceiling under the 1913 act was increased to 3,000 florins per year in 1941. This ceiling was much higher than those stipulated earlier in the statutes of the sickness funds. Thus, this increase was one of the greatest improvements of the 1941 decree. Dependents were also covered as a result of the 1941 decree and became indirectly insured.

Another improvement in the 1941 decree was that it brought uniformity and extended the benefits for the compulsorily insured (Ledeboer 1966, p. 9). It provided for medical care and a funeral benefit. There was no waiting period between joining the fund and receiving benefits, except for dental prostheses, nor were deductibles or co-payments charged, except for some forms of dental treatment and treatment in sanatoria. Contributions were calculated as a percentage of earnings, and one half was paid by the employer. These premiums were collected by the administrative bodies of the Sickness Act, that is, the occupational organizations and not the sickness funds. All these premiums were brought together in a mutual fund and were then distributed between the sickness funds according to need. Under the supervision provision, sickness funds wishing to be involved in the execution of the Sickness Funds Decree had to be recognized by the general secretary of social affairs. Moreover, a recognized sickness fund could not administer compulsory insurance programs unless it was approved by the general secretary. Such a fund (204 in all in 1941) (Ledeboer 1966, p. 9) was obliged to call itself a "general sickness fund." A recognized fund had to accept administrative and financial supervision by a "commissioner charged with the supervision of the sickness funds." Agreements between the funds and the providers had to be approved by this official.

Reactions to the Decree

According to De Vreeze, President of the National Hospital Council and member of Parliament, there was little reaction to the Sickness Funds Decree in the period 1940–1941, simply because, given wartime conditions, the parties involved had no opportunity to react. Reactions came when the war was over. According to Van den Berg, the former "commissioner charged with the supervision of the sickness funds," the Dutch physicians were disappointed by the government decision to maintain the 1941 decree after the war. They objected to the increase in the number of insured patients, and the resulting decrease in private practice (Van den Berg 1965, pp. 110–16). Furthermore, many opposed the state supervision of the sickness funds introduced by the decree (Van den Berg 1965, pp. 133–38). During the war, some thought had been given to the direction that Dutch health care policy would take once the country was liberated. The war ended in Europe on May 7, 1945. That summer, the Dutch Medical Association discussed its Health Care Organization Plan. This plan made a plea for a comprehensive health care policy, in which the function of the sickness funds would be limited to their original role of providing social insurance and they would have no responsibility for providing health care. The plan favored a balance among curative care, preventive care, and social hygiene and proposed the creation of a Department of Public Health at national level, equipped with statistical and research facilities. Implementation of the plan called for a new health professional—the public health officer—and new educational schemes for physicians and allied professions (Koninklijke Nederlandse Maatschappij 1946).

The 1967 Exceptional Medical Expenses Act

Insurance for Extended Care

The Netherlands came out of World War II with its physical assets badly damaged: its industrial plants, railroads, and bridges had been destroyed, and great parts of the country had been flooded. The country gradually recovered, helped by the Marshall Plan for Europe. Nevertheless, in the aftermath of the war, the Netherlands was confronted with serious problems in its large colonial territories in the Far East. Following a conflict that lasted several years, and competed for attention and energy with the task of rebuilding the homeland, these colonies cut themselves loose. In the health care field, through the 1964 Sickness Fund Act, the Government more or less confirmed the prevailing provisions of the Sickness Funds Decree introduced by the Germans in 1941. All wage earners and salaried workers with earnings below a stipulated ceiling were compulsorily insured for health care. Dependents and unemployed receiving unemployment cash benefits were also entitled to benefits in kind. The aged and their dependents could also join this scheme if their income did not exceed a given level. Benefits became more comprehensive: both general practitioner and specialist medical care; regular dental care check-ups; obstetric care; admission to hospitals and mental hospitals for periods up to one year; drugs and ambulance service.

The 1965 General Assistance Act, replacing the Poor Law, guaranteed indigent care to those who could not afford the cost of needed health care, or who could not afford to cover this risk by health insurance. The General Assistance Act provided in particular for inpatient treatment of mental patients and the care of the disabled. Furthermore, the municipalities, the administrative intermediaries of the General Assistance Act, could intervene to help meet the cost of long-term home care and the cost of individual health care not covered by health insurance. The self-employed and those wage and salary earners with an income above the ceiling stipulated for compulsory insurance were privately insured. These voluntary insurance schemes provided more or less the same benefits as the compulsory insurance scheme.

In 1962, the minister of public health had brought to the attention of the Social-Economic Council and the Central Council of Public Health the insufficient coverage by the prevailing sickness fund insurance for so-called "catastrophic" risks ("catastrophic" in the sense of a heavy financial burden), in his view the main problem of the national health efforts (Andriessen 1966, p. 71). For instance, the funds covered only 50 percent of the costs of extended care, for a maximum of one year per three-year period; acute hospital inpatient care was covered for a maximum of one year only; only 75 percent of costs for inpatient tuberculosis treatment was covered, though without time limit; and so on (Boer 1966, p. 498). Certain types of prolonged illness were not covered at all, for example, custodial or nursing home care for the physically or mentally handicapped. These last patients, a great many of them elderly cases of senile dementia, could seek care only through municipal authorities, within the General Assistance Act provisions for indigents, and subject to a means test (Sijses 1968, p. 11). According to the minister of public health, in his comments on the Exceptional Medical Expenses (EME) Bill introduced in 1965, the problems were important enough to justify legislative intervention because: everybody runs the risk of becoming a victim of prolonged illness, and practically no one can cope with the resulting financial implications; insurance on a voluntary basis had been proven incapable of meeting the costs of prolonged illness; and the existing situation was in flagrant contradiction with the principle of equity as a dominant social goal in Dutch society (Andriessen 1966, p. 71).

The 1967 Exceptional Medical Expenses Act in fact had many different origins. The starting point of the act's evolution was undoubtedly the widespread awareness of insufficient facilities for certain patient groups in Dutch society, especially, according to Querido, the young mentally retarded and the handicapped. A favorite example was the appalling shortage of facilities for senile dementia: for approximately 20,000 cases of senile dementia in the Netherlands in 1966, there were only 2,500 special beds.

This lack of special facilities was not regarded as a deficiency of the prevailing sickness fund insurance, since it was felt that the entire nation should contribute to facilities for these groups. The central question was how these risks, at that time insufficiently covered, could be more adequately covered by the nation as a whole. Since 1957 (when the General Pension Act was introduced), the Dutch had

had good experience with the concept of "people's insurance," a kind of social insurance that is not limited to wage and salary earners and their dependents, but which covers the entire population and is financed through special taxes, collected by the Internal Revenue Service, levied on all kinds of income (although only up to a certain ceiling). There was almost a universal feeling that this kind of social insurance offered a solution for the existing lack of special facilities for the mentally retarded, the handicapped, and the other under-served groups.

Although the problems of young mentally retarded and handi-capped persons stimulated the evolution of the Exceptional Medical Expenses Act, the problem of the aged, taken up and publicized by the two Dutch nursing home associations, ultimately dominated the issue. At this period, when appropriate institutions were lacking, married children who were not prepared to take care of their parents (as they had in the past) sent them to hospitals. From the early sixties, the nursing home associations (one without religious affiliation and the other Catholic) stressed that sick elderly people do not necessarily belong in hospitals, but rather in nursing homes. Nursing homes in the Netherlands are extended-care facilities for the aged. As a rule, these voluntary nonprofit organizations provide high standards of care. The nursing home associations argued that the elderly could be much better cared for in nursing homes than in general hospitals, and the care was also less expensive. An important element underlying this campaign was the fear that, if the elderly continued to be treated in hospital beds, hospitals would ultimately eliminate nursing homes altogether. Nursing home beds were scarce and financial resources to increase the number were lacking. So, the nursing home associations strongly backed the idea of the Excep-tional Medical Expenses Act, since it represented a sound basis for the required expansion of nursing home beds.

The Exceptional Medical Expenses Act further profited from the thriving economy of the mid-sixties, when money was easy to get and a collective building drive developed for the construction of roads, houses, community equipment, and health care institutions. The general feeling at the time was, that, notwithstanding the lip service paid to planning, it was better to build as much as possible; the government tacitly concurred.

Finally, there was a consensus in Dutch society that coverage of catastrophic risks should no longer be provided by the indigent care mechanism, but should be regarded as an automatic right of all Dutch inhabitants.

Reactions to the Bill

In the discussion concerning the Exceptional Medical Expenses Bill, there was some controversy about whether the government would limit its role to providing financial resources, or whether it should go a step further and enter into direct control of physical resources. The government's options were to build the required institutions itself or to rely on market forces for their development while regulating this development through a licensing system. Only one political party supported the first option, which regarded the Exceptional Medical Expenses Bill as a first step in the direction of a national health service on the British model (namely, the PSP, the Party of Pacifist Socialists). Virtually all the other political parties supported, with the minister, the second option, which they considered representative of the Dutch approach. In their mind the bill would provide a missing link, complementing the prevailing system of health care provision and completing a comprehensive, adequate system, accessible to all in need (Veldkamp 1967, p. 6). The bill was finally enacted through the normal Dutch legislative process. The majority of political parties supported the bill, as did concerned parties like hospital associations, nursing home associations, sickness funds, the Medical Association, and the commercial health insurance companies.

Scope and Content of the Act

The Exceptional Medical Expenses Act essentially mandates the financing, through earmarked general revenue, of long-term inpatient care, to be provided free at the time of service. However, some costs are shared by certain categories of patients, including: married insured patients of 18 years and older; married insured males of 18 years and older whose wives are also in institutions under the EME Act; and insured patients of 65 years and older. The amount of cost sharing varies according to the institution concerned and the insured's income. The underlying principle is that basic costs such as food and linen are in effect transferred from the home to the institution and should be covered by the patient from his normal income or from his pension. The scheme is financed partly by a special tax paid by all taxpayers. The government supplements the rest out of general revenue. The special tax is a percentage of all income, up to a certain ceiling (in 1973, 2.6 percent up to 24,300 florins, or $8,100). The taxes are collected by the Internal Revenue Service. In 1972, these taxes amounted to 1,370.8 million florins ($457 million, or 70 percent of the total fund) to which the state added 583.3 million florins ($194 million, or 30 percent). The taxes and the subsidy are pooled in a General Fund for Exceptional Medical Expenses, supervised by the Sickness Fund Council.

The Exceptional Medical Expenses Act covers the entire population, both residents and nonresidents (for example, migrant workers who are taxable in the Netherlands). The right to benefits is not linked to payment of the special tax, nor to health status. In principle, the right to benefits is in terms of need. Nonpayment of the special tax is a matter for the Internal Revenue Service. The main benefits of the Exceptional Medical Expenses Act in 1967 were, from the first day of need:

admission in extended-care facilities
admission in institutions for the mentally and physically handicapped
admission in institutions for the mentally retarded

and from the 366th day of need:

admission in acute hospitals and mental hospitals, the period before the 366th day being covered by the sickness fund insurance

According to Article 6 of the act, the sickness funds and commercial insurance companies are the carriers of the program. Because they do not have their own medical services, they contract with hospitals, nursing homes, and other institutions for the provision of care. The scheme is administered by a combination of agencies, namely, sickness funds, commercial health insurance companies, and the provincial institutes for health insurance of public employees. All are supervised by the Sickness Funds Council.

A Case of Indirect Development

With the introduction of this act, the government saw its specific role with respect to prolonged illness as one of providing sufficient financial resources to develop facilities for extended health care and for prolonged physical or mental illness. However, rather than establish a special development fund, these extended care facilities, including manpower, were to be developed by making coverage for this type of care possible—that is, by directing significant sums of money into this area of the health care delivery system. This idea was consistent with the opinion of the Central Council of Public Health, which had stated that the whole inpatient sector remained underdeveloped because insurance coverage was insufficient. Other authors predicted that implementation of the Exceptional Medical Expenses Act would indirectly stimulate development of the needed facilities (Verduyn 1966, p. 342).

However, the government did not intend to build or provide the needed facilities directly. It intended to rely on social and market forces, propelled by the substantial increase in financial resources that the act would make available. Some authors predicted that the Exceptional Medical Expenses Act would have a less desirable influence on the development of the total health care system. They warned that the emphasis on inpatient care would ultimately disrupt the balance between inpatient and outpatient care and would result in higher total health care costs (Minister van Sociale Zaken 1966, p. 284). Querido, a member of the First Chamber, voted against the act for this reason. But the minister and his state secretary did not share these doubts, since the act provided for a gradual introduction of social services and ambulatory care. A cost explosion, they argued, could be prevented by controlling tariffs and by the certification-of-need mechanism governing hospital construction. The minister was backed in his views by the Social-Economic Council; given the limited financial resources, coverage for inpatient care was considered as the first priority. Some forms of outpatient care could be covered afterwards, if inpatient care was shown to have caused unnecessary costs. The Council also proposed keeping hospital costs down by more stringent hospital admission criteria. All these arguments could not convince Querido. His point was that, in the absence of adequate ambulatory care provisions, referring physicians would have no other alternative than to send patients to an inpatient care facility (Dolman 1968, p. 65).

The 1974 Policy Proposal on the Structure of the Health Care System

Problems and Bottlenecks

During the most recent ten years, and particularly since the important 1966 Report on National Health Care and the introduction of the Exceptional Medical Expenses Act in 1967, health care has become a matter of great concern in the Netherlands. The 1973 government, in its statement of policy, considered "important reforms" in this area indispensable. The 1974 Policy Proposal on the Structure of the Health Care System indicates starting points for major reforms (on structure, functioning, financing, and so on) and their enactment through legislation. The 1974 Policy Proposal, however, is not a bill: its purpose is to stimulate discussion in Dutch society on health care matters. The proposal expresses concern about the growth of costs, and points out that although the Dutch health care system has a remarkable record compared to those of similar countries, it is nevertheless confronted by a series of problems and bottlenecks. Perceived against the background of rapidly increasing health care costs, the proposal lists the problems of the Dutch health care system as follows (Ministerie van Volksgezondheid 1974, p. 6):

1. Absense of cost-containment mechanisms, so that the costs of new developments in health care cannot be regulated or guided as rapidly as necessary.
2. Lack of integration of services, with the independent functioning of each component resulting in inefficient utilization of available manpower, equipment, and money, while the patient is overwhelmed by the system's complexity.
3. Limited direction through financing, because the system is financed from a wide range of sources and the financing mechanisms adapt passively to the changing needs of the prevailing organizational arrangements, with only a limited correcting effect on the integration of the system. In other words, financing is not used as a mechanism to reorient organizational arrangements.
4. Insufficient cooperation between social care and health care, which function independently, without an interface to evolve common policy on planning, financing, and other matters.
5. Dominance of hospital-based care, as a result of medico-technical developments and the financing mechanism of social insurance.

Inpatient care, in particular short-term general hospital care, had thus been allowed to develop almost without restraint, while ambulant, preventive, and mental health care remained underdeveloped.

6. Imbalances in the inpatient care sector itself, with shortages in some areas and overcapacity in others.

7. Problems of scale, in that the system contains oversized facilities which often function below their needed critical mass.

8. Uneven geographical distribution of services, particularly in mental health care.

9. Insufficient matching of manpower supply and health care needs.

10. Insufficient involvement of the health care consumer in the development and the functioning of the health care system.

A Blueprint for Change

The 1974 Policy Proposal has two main objectives. The first is to eliminate existing imbalances. In this sense, the proposal contains a number of sub-objectives corresponding to the listed problems. But, since the basic concern underlying the proposal is the health care cost explosion, its second objective is to contain costs within reasonable limits, without jeopardizing the health status achieved so far. In fact, this second objective overrides the first, since correction of the listed imbalances is proposed not only to improve function and integration, but also to contain costs. The two main principles proposed to change the health care delivery system are regionalization and structuring into echelons or levels of care (Ministerie van Volksgezondheid, 1974, p. 8).

Regionalization, as expressed in the Policy Proposal, means dividing the Netherlands into a number of health care regions, each providing within its boundaries a well-structured, comprehensive health care system (Ministerie van Volksgezondheid 1974, p. 10). The state secretary made this concept more specific in 1975 by designating five so-called experimental regions (Ministerie van Volksgezondheid September 1976). At that time he presented some details of his regionalization model and the strategy he wished to follow (Ministerie van Volksgezondheid October 1976). A democratically elected local and regional government, rather than a functional administrative hierarchy responsible only for health care matters, is

suggested. Whichever type of government is introduced, the decision-making agency should be democratically supervised and the
providers of health care should be involved in the decision-making
process through regional advisory committees. To support the
health care policy through a more integrated, regionally-oriented financing structure, a regional finance committee should be established. Another function to be performed at the regional level is
the supervision of the provision of health care. Data on capacity,
productivity, finance, and epidemiology should be collected at a central point in the region. The state secretary stressed that several
characteristics were important for the experimental regions:
regional budgeting; a regional authority structure, whether responsible for all regional matters, or focused exclusively on health care; a
regional institute for ambulatory mental health care; integration of
education and research in the provision of care; and integration of
health and social care. To stimulate and to develop the experiments,
200,000 fl per year ($66,667) were allocated.

Structuring into echelons or levels means grouping health care
into two echelons and then allocating manpower and facilities to the
respective echelons according to their degree of specialization (Ministerie van Volksgezondheid 1974, p. 11). The primary-care echelon
is to be organized around the general practitioner. Care is provided
mainly on an ambulatory basis, and the general practitioner cooper-
ates regularly with providers of social services. Settings for care are
group practices or neighborhood primary-care centers. The second
echelon, accessible in principle only via the primary-care level, contains specialist services structured into two main categories—somatic
care and mental health care—each of which includes ambulatory
and inpatient facilities (short- or long-term). Central to the idea of
structuring the health care system in these two echelons is the goal
of stressing the first echelon and minimizing the second one. This
reversal of well-known trends is dictated by the conviction that the
first echelon can cope adequately with problems now unnecessarily
dealt with in the second echelon. It is also hoped that primary care
will prove to be less expensive. Apart from the creation of two echelons for personal care, the 1974 proposal suggests the unification of
all public health activities into a single, so-called basic echelon, to be
responsible for all preventive measures directed towards the total
community and its environment (Ministerie van Volksgezondheid
1974, p. 18).

According to the 1974 Policy Proposal, the health care cost explosion in the Netherlands was caused by two developments: an increase in the prices of manpower and physical resources, and an increase in the volume of manpower and physical resources (Ministerie van Volksgezondheid 1974, p. 36). Together, between 1964 and 1974, these increases caused an average yearly cost increase of 18.5 percent. Thirteen percent of the yearly cost increase resulted from increasing prices of manpower and physical resources, while the remaining 5.5 percent yearly increase was caused by the increase in the volume of manpower and physical resources. More than one-half of this 5.5 percent increase, namely 3 percent, has been attributed to the Exceptional Medical Expenses Act while 1.3 percent resulted from population growth, and 1.2 percent from medical progress and quality improvement.

The influence of the 1967 Exceptional Medical Expenses Act on the increase in resources in the Netherlands is shown in the following figures:

	Number before the EME Act (1964)	Number after the EME Act (1969)	(1974)
extended-care beds	12,790	24,610	
beds for mentally retarded	15,940	20,330	
staff in extended-care facilities	9,800		34,100
staff in institutions for mentally retarded	10,700		18,100

The 1974 Policy Proposal suggests that the effect of the Exceptional Medical Expenses Act can be neutralized by reducing the capacity of the total inpatient care sector (except in some cases, such as provision for senile dementia) and by undertaking a restrained development of the primary-care echelon and public health efforts (Ministerie van Volksgezondheid 1974, p. 42). If cost containment is pursued through reduction of the volume of inpatient care provision, it will reinforce the need for changes in the delivery system. Indeed, a reduction of the bed/population ratio in general hospitals to 4:1,000 must be matched by an appropriate development of alternative modes of care, in particular at the primary-care level.

The implementation of the proposal's two main objectives, changing the delivery structure and containing costs, will be a long-term process, because the necessary legislation will have to be passed by Parliament. Two important bills deriving from the 1974 Policy Proposal, one related to the delivery structure (the Health Resources Bill), and the other concerning the prices in health care (the Health Care Tariffs Bill), were introduced in the Second Chamber in October 1976.

The Health Resources Bill (Ministrie van Volksgezondheid 1976, 14.181) aims at implementing rules to foster an efficient and effective health care delivery system. It reaffirms the Policy Proposal's statement that the central government is responsible for a well-structured, democratic, and adequate health care system, with the local and regional authorities acting in an advisory and executive capacity (Ministerie van Volksgezondheid 1974, p. 18). Health care planning becomes a responsibility at the subnational level, within the constraints posed by national guidelines. The Policy Proposal did not clarify whether the subnational authorities responsible for health would be created ad hoc or whether the existing civil authorities, regional and local, would have responsibility. The bill leaves no doubt in favoring the latter.

The Health Care Tariffs Bill (Ministerie van Volksgezondheid 1976, 14.182) was introduced to implement a new, threefold financing structure, suggested in the Policy Proposal, to correspond to the new delivery structure envisioned. The basic echelon, or public health care echelon, is to be financed from general revenue. The primary-care level, including the Cross Organizations (private organizations involved mainly in home care and preventive health care, which are now mainly financed by subsidies and contributions of their membership) are to be financed through social security contributions. The secondary-care level is also to be financed through social security contributions. Moreover, the bill aims at containing health care costs by increasing government involvement in the tariff negotiations between health care providers and sickness funds. In principle, both partners, the providers and the funds, will retain initiative in proposing tariffs. However, these tariffs will have to be approved by a new government body; the Central Agency for Health Care Tariffs, which will replace the Central Agency for Hospital Tariffs and, to a certain extent, the Sickness Fund Council. The minister of public health, together with his colleagues in the departments of economic and social affairs, can issue guidelines to this agency. If the two primary interested parties cannot reach an agreement on the tariffs, the Central Agency itself will determine them, in accordance with the ministerial guidelines. The secretary of state reckons that by containing the volume of resources and by controlling the tariffs in health care, he can control costs (since they consist of volume multiplied by prices). If passed, the bills will pave the way for a regionalized, balanced, and cost-containable health care delivery system. Meanwhile, several short-term measures related to the Policy Proposal are under way. As mentioned above, in October 1975 the State Secretary designated five regions for experimentation in health care matters:

Nijmegen. In this region, the experiment will focus on the coordination of admission and discharge policies in somatic as well as mental health care institutions, to develop a clearer view of the feasibility and functioning of the proposed echelon structure.

Maastricht. A medical school was recently established in this region, and it is hoped to develop effective links with the regional health care system. Therefore, special attention is to be paid to the integration of medical education and research in the provision of health care. Another task is the analysis of the region's health care costs, to discover whether the regional cost structure fits in with existing national health care financing structures. Opportunities to develop an integrated information system in the region are also to be investigated.

Friesland. During the experiment, special attention will be paid to the integration of social care, health care, and the district health care services as they are already functioning in this region.

Kennemerland. Special attention will be paid here to reducing the emphasis on inpatient care in favor of ambulatory and primary care.

Eindhoven. The experiment will focus in this region on the duties, functions and responsibilities of the projected regional authorities, taking into account the present responsibilities of the municipalities. The result of the experiment should indicate to what extent legislative action is required.

In addition to the regional experiments, two other short-term measures are to be implemented. The first is the installation of pilot organizations and pilot groups for clearly defined projects and for the development of neighborhood primary-care centers (Ministerie van Volksgezondheid, 1974, p. 43); directly related to the Policy Proposal is the so-called Provisional Regulation for the Development of

Experimental Neighborhood Health Centers of July 3, 1974 (Ministerie van Cultuur 1974). The second measure is the reduction of the bed/population ratio for general hospitals from 5.4 to 4.0 per 1,000 inhabitants (Ministerie van Volksgezondheid 1974, p. 43).

Positions of the Interest Groups

The Dutch Medical Association (Koninklijke Nederlandse Maatschappij 1974) regrets the absence in the Policy Proposal of measures regarding occupational health care; it objects to priorities based on cost containment, which could be achieved by other means, like efficient utilization of available manpower and other resources, substitution for expensive services of equally effective but less expensive ones, and so on. Moreover, the proposed cost-containing measures will, the association argues, jeopardize the present standard of care.

The 1974 Policy Proposal emphasizes the dominant role of the central government in defining Dutch health care policy. The Dutch Medical Association rejects, however, any system in which the providers of care are only involved at the executive level and left out of the decision-making process. Further, the association does not agree with the opinion expressed in the Policy Proposal that outpatient care has remained underdeveloped because of an overdeveloped inpatient care sector. Moreover, it doubts that a reinforced primary-care sector will automatically diminish the demand for inpatient care facilities. Finally, the association has reacted negatively to both of the recent bills based on the Policy Proposal. A special general assembly, held in mid-February 1977, rejected the health resources bill on the grounds that it does not involve providers of care in decision-making. As for the health care tariffs bill, the physicians agree with the principle of limiting incomes only if it is applied to workers in all sectors.

The National Hospital Council (Nationale Ziekenhuis Raad 1974), as the representative organization of all the Dutch inpatient care institutions, wants to preserve the role played by private initiative. It considers the proposed levels, or echelons, too rigid. On the one hand, they do not take into account the different specialties already existing at the first level, while on the other hand the proposed structure overlooks the fact that general hospitals are increasingly involved with primary care through outpatient services. Hospital planning cannot continue to be based, as in the past, on the number of hospital beds, because this notion does not encompass a realistic view of hospital outpatient and inpatient functions. The council considers the Policy Proposal to be ruinous for the inpatient sector in particular, and for the quality of Dutch health care in general. According to the council, the creation of a government-organized information system, added to the systems that have already been developed through private initiative (and which are not reluctant to share data with the government), would be useless. Up to now, the Council has published no official reaction to the health resources and health care tariffs bills.

Human Resources

Health Manpower

In the Netherlands there is a prevailing opinion that, with regard to health manpower development, the 1941 Sickness Funds Decree indirectly reinforced the position of the general practitioner, much as the 1911 National Insurance Act did in Britain. But quantitative evidence for this belief is lacking. In contrast, the effects of the Exceptional Medical Expenses Act on health manpower development could be calculated. Generally speaking, health manpower development was not included in the health insurance scheme of 1941, nor in its reform in 1967. Human resources in the Netherlands have instead developed according to a pattern in which private initiative and government share responsibility for the development. This pattern is true for all types of health manpower: physicians, allied health professions, and the recently created health care managers.

Professional organizations represent private initiative. Professional organizations of physicians, dental surgeons, pharmacists, nurses, and others have consistently been concerned with the quantity and the quality of the groups they represent and have initiated regulations on both aspects. After some time, the government has usually approved these regulations, although to varying degrees.

In 1932 the Dutch Medical Association initiated the Medical Specialist Registration, which led to long discussions with the government on the issue of specialist qualifications. These in turn resulted in two commissions—the Central Council and the Specialist Registration Committee—which determine the training requirements for certification as a specialist and supervise the fulfillment of these requirements (Querido 1973, p. 145). Because these commissions were created with full government involvement, the government felt no need for special legislation in the area. The government did initiate some legislation on the spatial distribution of physicians during the war. An act passed in September 1939 stated that physicians could be appointed to replace drafted colleagues, while the establishment of a new medical practice was subject to approval by the State Inspectorate (Querido 1965, p. 192).

As recently as 1975, the physicians' professional associations showed evidence of their continuing commitment to manpower development. In that year, the Dutch General Practitioners' Association, a subdivision of the Dutch Medical Association, put forward a policy plan containing a general practitioner distribution proposal (Landelijke Huisartsen Vereniging 1975). The plan links a spatial distribution policy and a policy to reduce the size of general practitioners' practices. The General Practitioners' Association proposes to limit the number of insured patients (and consequently of all patients) inscribed on a general practitioner's list from 3,000 to 2,500 within four years. Being a guideline, this limitation does not automatically apply to every region in the country. A regional committee of the General Practitioners' Association can make the maximum figure applicable at the request of a general practitioner who is already practicing in a region, or at the request of a general practitioner wanting to practice there. The decision can be appealed to a national committee by the general practitioner involved, the local sickness fund, the State Inspectorate, or all the general practitioners in the region. If the maximum figure is made applicable to a certain region at a particular general practitioner's request, he is obliged to compensate other general practitioners' financially for their loss of patients. This kind of policy, known as "supported free establishment," should make possible a real general practitioners distribution policy. A chart indicating "open" areas would have to be updated once or twice a year.

The Dutch General Practitioners' Association, being the general practitioners' representative organization, feels more or less obliged to promote a distribution policy, because otherwise the government itself would push it. In fact, a new trend is emerging in the pattern of shared responsibility for manpower development. Whereas in the past the government adopted practices initiated by private organizations only gradually, it has recently begun to play a much more active role; if private initiative wants to maintain its leading position, it will have to act more vigorously. This change was already apparent to a certain extent in the 1966 Report on National Health Care (Ministerie van Sociale Zaken 1966, p. 166). In this document, the government expressed the belief that its role was to improve the quality of care by improving the continuing education and raising the standards of education and training for health care providers. Further, it would increase the quantity of health manpower, for example, by establishing a new medical school in Rotterdam.

The shift to greater government action is even more obvious in the 1974 Policy Proposal, which states that "manpower planning—as part of overall planning—covering all qualitative and quantitative aspects, is necessary" (Ministerie van Volksgezondheid 1974, p. 27). Obviously, such manpower planning poses many problems; for example, new roles and divisions of tasks will have to be defined within new organizational settings and group practices, and a long period will be required to adjust the manpower supply because educational schemes involve from six to ten years (although the proposal includes retraining and special continuing education for health workers as a partial solution to this problem).

The 1974 Policy Proposal expresses deep concern about the future number of general practitioners and medical specialists, since uncontrolled increases would, according to the state secretary, result in another cost explosion because of an expanded number of initiators of costly diagnostic and other interventions. Moreover, increases beyond a certain doctor/population ratio do not necessarily improve the quality of health care. Taking current rates of population growth and medical manpower increase, the proposal projects an approximate ratio of 1.8 physicians per 1,000 inhabitants by 1982. Thus, while the 1966 report simply acknowledged a lack of physicians and indicated some occasional solutions, the 1974 proposal considers the government's responsibility for human resources development as part of its general responsibility for an efficient and effective health care system: "Of great importance to the controllability of health care is the quantitative aspect of available manpower, in particular the number of general practitioners and specialists" (Ministerie van Volksgezondheid 1974, p. 28).

The Health Care Resources Bill introduced in October 1976 puts forward concrete legislation to implement the 1974 Policy Proposal. Chapter 5 of the bill contains measures that will eventually enable the government to match the supply and distribution of health workers to the required number and distribution emerging from the regional and local health care plans, designed by the regional and local authorities according to guidelines put forward by the central government. To begin, establishment of free-practicing health workers will be discouraged indirectly through a licensing system. The sickness funds will be unable to make a contract with a health worker unless he or she is licensed by the government. If not licensed, the health worker will be limited to private practice, which, in view of the modest income prospects from the small group of voluntary insured, should be unattractive.

In a second stage, this licensing system will be replaced by a certification-of-need system. In this system, practice as a health worker, throughout the whole country or in a part of the country, will depend on government permission. The bill also empowers the government to limit the size of existing practices and to instruct closer cooperation among free-practicing health workers and health care institutions. The bill empowers the secretary of state to lay down quality requirements relating, for example, to the organization and administration of a practice. If these requirements are not met, a license or permit to practice can be refused or revoked. While this bill is still in Parliament, earlier measures giving government legislative control over physician development have already been enacted. An act of 1970, reaffirmed and partially changed in 1972 and 1975, gives the minister of education the power to limit the intake of students in medical schools, which in turn affects the number of physicians eventually at work in the Netherlands. Since then, only a fixed number of students have been permitted to enter the medical schools. This measure evolved apart from the 1974 Policy Proposal, although the proposal does approve it. In fact, this act had been envisaged for some time. Between 1930 and 1940, different interest groups had urged the government to diminish the number of physicians by limiting the number of medical students. In 1931, a state commission headed by Zeegers advised the government to close the Medical School at Groningen (Huysmans 1973, p. 168). Two years later, another state commission, headed by Limburg, recommended limiting the number of students, and in 1939 the Dutch Medical Association made a similar proposal (Van Es 1968, p. 109).

The pattern of dual responsibility also applies to health professionals other than physicians, such as nurses and pharmacists.

Schemes for the training of nurses and other allied professions were primarily initiated by their professional organizations. After some years, the government supported these schemes while requiring, in turn, certain quality standards. This policy resulted quite early (1921) in the legal protection of the Diploma of Nursing (Ministerie van Sociale Zaken 1966, p. 29). Another example is the distribution policy for Dutch pharmacists initiated (years ago) by the Dutch Pharmacists' Association. This policy had two purposes: to guarantee each pharmacist an adequate population base and to rationalize the distribution of pharmacists by dividing the country into pharmacy areas. This system is still in operation, although since 1958 the government has shared responsibility for the determination of the pharmacy areas (Ministerie van Sociale Zaken 1966, p. 29).

In relation to these allied professionals, too, the government did make some early initiatives. Querido cites an effort to promote the development of new types of health workers. In 1925 the government established a State Commission on Maternity Care, which defined three new health professions and proposed a very detailed plan for their education and licensing. As Querido points out, it is remarkable that the commission did not even consider how to pay for this education, or how the new workers would be remunerated. Furthermore, the plans were never enacted (Querido 1965, p. 172). More recently, however, the government has taken a more active part in the training schemes for allied health professions. The 1976 budget for public health and environmental hygiene provides 17,686,300 florins ($5,895,000) to subsidize educational schemes of more than ten allied professions.

The situation with regard to health care managerial manpower is slightly different, probably because health care managers have only recently been recognized as a category of health manpower. Up to 1974, the Dutch government did little with regard to the quality and quantity of managerial resources, although one of the policy goals of the 1966 report was to pay more attention to the education of hospital managers. The 1974 Policy Proposal did not touch on the subject, although in the public debate on the Policy Proposal in the Second Chamber in mid-1975 the state secretary declared that he recognized a need for the training and continuing education of health care managers. He also declared himself in favor of the idea of a national "school of public health," although this idea remains under discussion (Staatssecretaris Hendriks 1975, p. 702).

In the meantime, the universities took the initiative. From 1960 to 1971, the Netherlands' only operational program devoted to part-time training in hospital and health services administration was at the University of Tilburg. The courses offered in this program are more accurately described as continuing education than as degree courses, because they build on the experience of practicing administrators who continue to fulfill their managerial responsibilities while spending a limited time, spread over nine months, in the training institution (World Health Organization 1972, p. 9).

In 1969, at the University of Amsterdam, the Institute for Hospital Sciences was founded. The objectives of this institute are to plan the new academic health sciences center at the University of Amsterdam, to provide graduate education in health services management, and to support health services research. At the University of Utrecht, a similar Institute for Hospital Sciences was created in 1970, with the objectives of providing education in health services management at the graduate level, and undertaking health services research (Blanpain and Delesie 1976, p. 394). Programs for training in hospital and health services administration are being developed at both universities, in connection with the development of these institutes for hospital sciences (World Health Organization 1972, p. 21). Several other educational institutions have followed suit: the Technical University of Eindhoven, which graduated its first health care industrial engineers in 1973; the technical universities of Delft and Twente, where doctoral students have worked on the application of industrial engineering to hospital problems; and the Higher School for Health Care of Utrecht, which in 1974 initiated an experimental schema to train health education consultants (Ministerie van Financiën 1976, p. 36).

Health Consumers

In the Netherlands, as in most other West European countries, the status of consumers in the health care system is related to the system of payment for health care through a variety of sickness funds. Although at the beginning there were numerous local organizations (650 in 1920), often dealing with health consumers on an individual basis, they have progressively merged and reduced in number, so that in 1976 there were only eighty. Thus, although they may originally have provided an important way for the consumer to express complaints or to influence policy, they are no longer able to fulfill such a function effectively.

On the other hand, the Netherlands is not immune to the consumer pressures developing in most Western countries as the result of highly professionalized and increasingly expensive health care systems. Indeed, the 1974 Health Care Policy Proposal includes a specific section on "democratization." However, the language is vague, and no specific proposals are listed for implementing consumer influence. Two organizations in the Netherlands are extremely interested in the promotion of health care consumerism: The Consumentenbond is an organization based in The Hague that is similar to the American Consumers' Union. It responded to the 1974 Policy Proposal by urging a much more definitive role for the consumer. Werkgroep 2000 is a voluntary organization in Amersfoort devoted to futurology, supported in part by funds from the national government. The health care section, under the direction of Dr. A. H. J. Thiadens, has been very active in developing new and more democratic concepts of health care organization. The current live issues in consumerism may be classified as follows:

1. Consumer and patient education. Most efforts by health departments, schools and disease-related organizations like the Diabetesvereniging are of a traditional sort. The Consumentenbond has published studies on health insurance, physician fees, drug prices and waiting times in clinics.
2. Patients' rights and the handling of grievances. Two or three hospitals have now appointed ombudsmen, and the Werkgroep 2000 is publicizing the Patients' Bill of Rights of the American Hospital Association. Professor J. F. Rang, a lawyer by training, has been appointed Professor of Health Rights at the University of Leiden Faculty of Medicine.
3. Participation by organized consumers and patients in the health care system. This is still a fragmentary movement, and has not been implemented by the government at all. However, a psychiatric hospital in the Province of Utrecht, the Willem Arntsz Ziekenhuis, now has a patients' parliament, democratically organized. The president of the parliament has the right to confer with the hospital's administrator and to provide patient input for management decisions.

In summary, although the consumer role in health care in the Netherlands is still modest, there are several indications that it will rapidly increase in the next decade.

Physical Resources

Hospitals

Before World War II, the government relied completely upon social forces (deriving mainly from private organizations and groups) for the development of health care institutions. A limited number of municipalities built their own hospitals because the Poor Law required them to provide for the health of the poor (Ministerie van Sociale Zaken 1966, p. 22). The majority of health care institutions, however, were owned by private organizations. By 1940, some academics and health care officials realized that the market forces had caused a kind of erratic, patchwork development. This awareness—though not general—led to a plan to regulate the building of new hospitals, through a certification-of-need system, and to establish a hospital board, with representatives from private organizations and government (Querido 1965, p. 182). But these plans were never implemented. Sometimes initiatives could not be enforced for lack of supporting legislation. For example, from 1920 the inspectors of the State Inspectorate had advisory responsibilities with respect to the building or renewal of hospitals. However, their advice, having no compelling character, could be ignored, and often was.

During the war the 1941 Sickness Funds Decree was introduced. As with human resources, its consequences on the development of physical resources are difficult to measure, and the extent to which it was responsible for the hospital boom of the first decade after the war is difficult to estimate. According to Dr. Marselis of the Sickness Fund Council, the decree's influence on hospital building only took hold in 1950. He believes that the boom between 1945 and 1950 was caused by reconstruction measures and expanded construction.

Thus, between 1945 and 1967, the Dutch government had no legal instruments to influence the development of physical resources in a direct way. But the Reconstruction Act did offer an indirect approach. To stimulate the rebuilding of destroyed hospitals, the Department of Reconstruction could act as loan guarantors for private organizations. Because the state could act as guarantor, the organizations could borrow money at a lower rate of interest. Through this guarantee system, the government had the opportunity to influence the building of hospitals, since it could refuse the guarantee if it considered the proposed hospital unnecessary. However, this was not really a very effective way to control development. If refused a loan, a private organization could always borrow money at a higher rate in the usual capital market, and therefore bypass the Reconstruction Department's restrictions. Nevertheless, once a private organization had accepted the State's guarantee, the State Building Service of the Department of Home Affairs had considerable control over the building of that specific institution, and even the color of the tiles did not escape the Department's eye. The guarantee system of the Reconstruction Act was abolished in 1967.

The 1967 Exceptional Medical Expenses Act was important for the development of the physical resources for health care in the Netherlands. By making possible the coverage of so-called catastrophic risks, the government hoped to encourage an increase in nursing homes and other facilities for prolonged physical or mental illness.

For actual building, the government continued to rely on market forces, and all the important groups supported the government in this point of view. The government did, however, feel the need to regulate such "spontaneous" activity (which was, in fact stimulated mainly by feeding considerable amounts of money into this area of the delivery system) through a licensing system. Article 8 of the Exceptional Medical Expenses Act required that every institution wishing to be eligible for the money made available through the act be licensed by the minister of health. The minister saw his role, through licensing, as one of guaranteeing acceptable quality and adequate territorial distribution. However, at the beginning he overestimated the potential of the market to cope with an enormous demand, because the shortage of facilities, in particular nursing homes and institutions for mentally retarded, persisted despite a rapid increase in the number of beds. This forced him, shortly after introduction of the act, to grant licenses to facilities of varying quality.

As time went by, however, institutions were built and renewed to meet higher standards. The licensing became very stringent, and patients treated in nonlicensed institutions faced a problem if they wished to have their costs reimbursed (*Sociale Verzekeringswetten*, p. 123). (In this, however, the Minister was apparently more anxious about the economic situation of the country than about the quality of care.) At the end of the sixties, the Netherlands still lacked a legal instrument for the explicit planning of the supply of health care institutions. In 1966 a certification-of-need system was suggested. This certification-of-need system was different from the licensing system of the Exceptional Medical Expenses Act. Where a certification-of-need system does not necessarily pay attention to quality, the Dutch licensing system had taken quality standards into account.

The certification-of-need system was embodied in the 1971 Hospital Provision Act (Wet 25 maart 1971), but this act turned out to be a dead letter, apart from a few articles (2; 23; 27; 29; 30) that established the Council for Hospital Provisions and brought into effect some transitional provisions. In September 1976, however, as a cost-containing measure, the state secretary introduced a certification-of-need system for expensive equipment in hospitals and for new specialist positions on hospital staffs. The measure has been justified as an implementation of Article 18.2 of the 1971 act, but the Dutch Medical Association, the Dutch Medical Specialists' Association, and the National Hospital Council object to this measure as being illegal (Koninklijke Nederlandse Maatschappij 1976; Nationale Ziekenhuis Raad 1976).

The main purpose of the 1971 act, the creation of a single national hospital plan, was never achieved. Fully aware that the act was not workable, the state secretary of public health proposed amendments to the act, focusing on the planning process, hospital closure, and the establishment of a liquidation fund (Ministerie van Volksgezondheid October 1974).

The planning process. The planning procedure outlined in the 1971 act required the drafting of a single overall national hospital plan targeted for a given date and based on the different provincial hospital plans. Thus, this national plan had to indicate the need for hospitals of all categories for the entire country; but, as the state secretary argued, such a task would require a series of decisions that are difficult to accomplish at any one moment. Moreover, in a continuously changing society, he stated, a planned end result is almost impossible to achieve. At least partly for this reason, the 1971 act remained largely inoperative.

The State Secretary suggested that the emphasis in the planning process should not be on the end result, but on the process itself, through the continuing adaptation of the plan to changed circumstances. To this end, greater differentiation in the planning process was proposed: the national hospital plan ought to be built upon a series of minor plans, each one concerning one special category of facilities, one special region, or even one special facility in one special region. The advantage of these minor plans was that they would be easier to prepare. A minor plan that had already been approved. could later be changed to fit another approved minor plan. The responsibility for the overall plan would rest upon the minister of public health. Normally, the minor plans would be drawn up by the regional authorities. But the minister would have the opportunity to influence the details of the minor plans, in cooperation with the regional authorities.

Hospital closure. The possibility that the need for hospital facilities in a given region might be less than the facilities already provided was not considered in the 1971 Hospital Provision Act. According to the state secretary, the establishment of an efficient health care structure requires the legal power to close hospitals or parts of them when they no longer fit in with the overall hospital plan. Furthermore, the minister should have the authority to close hospitals in the interests of quality of care. In such cases, the closing of hospitals could be implemented through the licensing system of the 1964 Sickness Fund Act and the 1967 Exceptional Medical Expenses Act. Obviously, such dramatic measures should only be taken with the full knowledge of the concerned hospital and regional authorities. Further, the advice of the Council for Hospital Provisions would have to be sought.

Liquidation Fund. In some cases, hospital authorities might agree that their hospital ought to be closed, but their final decision would be inhibited for financial reasons. Therefore, the establishment of a liquidation fund was proposed. A voluntary closing would have to be approved by the minister before the fund could intervene. The fund could also intervene in cases of compulsory closing.

The National Hospital Council and the Council for Hospital Provisions, an official council created by the 1971 Hospital Provision Act, were invited to comment on these three amendments. Whereas the National Hospital Council was not convinced of the necessity of changing the act (Nationale Ziekenhuis Raad 1975), the Council for Hospital Provisions agreed that changes were required because of changed views on the planning process, as reflected in the amendments (College voor Ziekenhuisvoorzieningen 1975). Another reason for changing the existing Hospital Provision Act was the state secretary's widely publicized intention to reduce general hospital beds to four per thousand population. In anticipation of such a reduction, a 1971 government measure had already delayed the building of new health care institutions. On February 13, 1975, this measure was replaced by a measure stipulating only 500,000,000 florins ($160,000,000) as the sum available for the building of health care institutions (Ministerie van Financiën 1976, p. 24). This amount only covers the building costs and does not include money for equipment, heating, electricity supply, and so on. Parliament began debate on this amendment to the 1971 Hospital Provision Act in February 1977, and the amendment was approved in the Second Chamber very quickly.

Once enacted, the amended 1971 act will be replaced by the comprehensive Health Resources Act, if the bill passes Parliament. There is a growing awareness that a comprehensive health care system cannot be provided through rigidly categorized instruments like the Hospital Provision Act. The Health Resources Bill contains statutory regulations to guarantee that the health services (Ministerie van Volksgezondheid 1976, 14181): (1) form a system with a clear but flexible structure; (2) function within this system in close interrelation; (3) are oriented towards providing a certain standard of quality of care; (4) are quantitatively controllable; and (5) furnish the necessary data for research and evaluation.

Looking backward, analysis shows that, whereas up to the mid-sixties there were no legal tools to influence directly the development of physical resources, this situation changed through the 1967 Exceptional Medical Expenses Act and the 1971 Hospital Provision Act; and it will change even more radically through the amended Hospital Provision Act and its probable successor, the Health Resources Act.

In one area, the prewar mechanism for the development of physical resources has not changed at all, nor can changes be expected in the immediate future: namely, the reliance upon market forces for the actual development of physical resources. However, the government attitude in this area is no longer passive, as it was in the past. If the government considers a certain development initiated as a result of social forces to be undesirable, either quantitatively or qualitatively, it has, and in the future will have increasingly, the opportunity to discourage this development. On the other hand, if it considers such a development conducive to the quality of care, it can stimulate it.

Health Centers

A recent example of a legal tool available for stimulating the development of health care facilities is the Provisional Regulation for the Development of Experimental Neighborhood Health Centers of 1974 (Ministerie van Cultuur 1974). Through this regulation, the state secretary of public health, together with the minister of culture, recreation, and social work, hopes to encourage three trends in Dutch health care: an increase in general practitioners seeking to cooperate—in different ways—with other general practitioners and health workers to improve their own working conditions and the quality of care; a desire on the part of public health nurses to break out of their isolation by teaming up with other health and social care workers; and a growing consensus that different modes of care and services should be offered "under the same roof" in health centers, service centers, and similar facilities.

To support these trends, the state secretary of public health and his colleague, the minister of culture, recreation, and social work, decided to promote the establishment of neighborhood health centers by means of a temporary granting policy. A neighborhood health center is described as "A permanent cooperative relationship between general practitioner(s), public health nurse(s) and social worker(s), having at their disposal a central address for advice and help and adequate facilities, and all serving the same population group." To be eligible for grants, a neighborhood health center must include at least two general practitioners, two public health nurses, and one social worker. Other professionals, such as obstetricians, psychologists, and pharmacists, can also be subsidized as part of the team.

One of the most important problems confronting the neighborhood health centers in the Netherlands is their financing. An overall and balanced coverage of all costs would require fundamental changes in the payments made by the sickness funds insurance and in the present method of governmental support of the Cross Organizations and the social service agencies. However, the development of neighborhood health centers cannot be delayed simply because the financing methods need to be overhauled; therefore, as part of the provisional regulation, the state secretary drafted a provisional financing method to compensate health centers for the extra cost resulting from the shift towards cooperative provision of primary-care services. This compensation consists of yearly grants, for a period of not more than five years, up to a maximum of 6,000 florins per year ($2,000) per employee. Social workers are eligible for subsidies only if they have been transferred on a temporary basis to the neighborhood health center from the social service agencies for which they originally worked. The entire grant is paid by the Ministry of Public Health, which recovers the amount allocated for social workers from the Ministry of Social Work.

In the provisional regulation, the state secretary for public health also announced the establishment of a national coordinating committee to advise on the preparation of projects, to stimulate the exchange of experience, and to evaluate the results of new working methods and relations. He further established a committee to advise on the performance of the provisional regulation, and to follow up the development of subsidized neighborhood health centers. This committee includes representatives from private organizations and civil servants from the two ministries involved. In an explanatory note to the 1976 budget for Public Health and Environmental Hygiene, the state secretary said that the provisional regulation had to be applied in a flexible way. The main criterion for awarding grants is the existence of formal modes of cooperation between health professionals (Ministerie van Financiën 1976, p. 726). In 1975, thirty neighborhood health centers received grants under the terms of the provisional regulation, while in 1974 only fourteen had (Ministerie van Financiën 1976, p. 27).

Other Facilities

The 1974 policy proposal devotes considerable attention to the development of mental health facilities. The proposal contains detailed plans for ambulatory mental health care, including regional institutes from which all ambulatory mental health care in a region would be organized and which would further cooperate with inpatient care facilities, social services, and community services. Inpatient care for mental patients would be provided in three settings: psychiatric hospitals, psychiatric departments in general hospitals, and special psychogeriatric institutions. There is still a significant shortage of such facilities in the Netherlands, especially for psychogeriatric patients. Also, a great number of general hospitals still lack psychiatric wards. The proposal acknowledges that the mental health policy is somewhat in conflict with the thrust of the rest of the proposal, since, while the proposal basically proposes to contain future expenditure, it calls for major expenditure to implement its mental health objectives (Ministerie van Volksgezondheid 1974, p. 48). Preventive health care facilities have developed through two stages. In the first stage, private organizations took initiatives (for example, in public health nursing and tuberculosis control), which were later supported by the government. This usually occurred spontaneously, although in some cases the government urged one or another private organization to take an initiative. The policy of government support involved more than giving money. For example, public health nursing was financed only if it included tuberculosis control. This required given qualifications, given education and educational programs, and so on. Despite this financial assistance, however, the government had no firm control over the quality of the preventive services themselves. This lack of quality control was one of the reasons for a shift from a policy of subsidies to a policy of using health insurance as the mechanism to implement given preventive programs. This shift represents the second stage in preventive facilities developments.

During the decade 1960–1970, a number of preventive activities that had originally received direct government support were brought under the health insurance scheme, and thus under the licensing system. The community mental health centers are a recent example of this development. Other reasons for this shift from a subsidy policy to an insurance policy were the desire to eliminate annual budget submissions and the desire to create a single, integrated finance system. The granting policy has led to what Querido described to us as a "tripartite responsibility":

1. The government has responsibility for providing sufficient financial resources. This does not mean, however, that all these resources come out of general revenue.
2. Private organizations have responsibility for distributing these resources among the groups whose interests they represent.
3. The individual citizen is responsible for an efficient use of the allocated resources.

Information Resources

Health Research

Health research in the Netherlands has historically been the prerogative of the universities. Although they are almost entirely funded by the Ministry of Education, even including their teaching hospitals, they have nevertheless operated quite independently of the ministry. This independence, quite understandably, has inhibited efforts to streamline health research and bring it in line with national priorities on health and health services. Two deliberate efforts have recently been made to reorient health research.

The first effort, initiated by the Ministry of Education, actually consists of two approaches. The first approach involves the creation of nationwide university institutes. The lack of a national research policy, and the impossibility of imposing such a policy upon the universities if it did exist, made government aware of the need for a mechanism to generate a coordinated research policy automatically. Thus, it was thought that a network of long-term associations between departments from different universities with separate and independent boards would result in more coherent research efforts. Although these interuniversity institutes are primarily funded by the Ministry of Education, they can also apply for funds from other sources. These institutes have already produced more coordinated health research and results of a higher quality than would have been possible without them, in biomedical as well as in health services research.

The second approach within the Ministry of Education involves the Organization for the Advancement of Pure Research, which has a branch dealing with health research called the Foundation for Medical Research. The organization was created in 1950 to direct basic research through a specifically created financing mechanism. The financing mechanism involves special grants towards specific "research communities," which consist of cooperative groups of individual researchers active in a specific area of medicine. The small grants are intended primarily as seed money, to encourage the individual researchers to mobilize other financial resources, such as university funds, towards specific projects. Important biomedical research in the Netherlands in the areas of cell genetics, cardiac function, immunopathology, and steroid hormones has been stimulated through this program.

The second effort to bring about a reorientation of health research started within the Ministry of Public Health and Environmental Hygiene. Again two approaches can be identified. The first approach involves the Netherlands Organization for Applied Scientific Research (TNO). Founded in 1932, this organization runs several institutes and laboratories. It is funded by those ministries involved with the relevant research areas, and it is governed by a board that includes scientists as well as representatives from the particular ministries. The Ministry of Public Health and Environmental Hygiene is the TNO's main source of funding. In 1970, a Council for Health Research was created within TNO with a view to setting priorities in health research. Specific institutes of the TNO are concerned with preventive medicine, radiology, experimental gerontology, and medical physics. Within the TNO and the Council for Health Research, there is a Committee on the Organization and Functioning of the Health Care System, which is charged with coordinating and supervising the research projects of both the TNO and the Council for Health Research.

The second approach of the Ministry of Public Health and Environmental Hygiene is the direct funding of specific research projects pertaining to national health problems. These direct grants have gained importance recently, because of the ministry's growing control over health services development and the widely felt need for mission-oriented health research relevant to national problems. Two recent projects are important with respect to health resources development. One is the development of a macroeconometric model of the health care sector, with a cross-sectional analysis aimed at measuring demand-supply elasticities in all types of health care delivery systems (Hulten, Van der Gaag, and Van Praag 1975). The second project is the development of a hospital costing model on the basis of hospital input variables (Groot et al. 1974, 1975). These direct grants for mission-oriented research projects are primarily responsible for the development of a systems-oriented, higher-level health research policy, and its implementation, in the Netherlands. Furthermore, this development is enhanced by the overlap of many advisory councils at the national level, in the research institutions themselves, and even at the level of individual research projects. Indeed, systems-oriented, higher-level research projects have proven inevitable in the attempt to solve real-life problems. The Hospital Provision Act, which was oriented exclusively around bed ratios, is a good example how a too simplistic approach proved unworkable when real-life problems had to be solved; a much more refined and complex methodology emerged as the only realistic approach.

The recent designation by the Ministry of Public Health and Environmental Hygiene of five experimental regions with special responsibilities in the development of a feasible national short- and long-term health policy also proves the point that future research must be increasingly mission-oriented. In prescribing the duties and providing subsidies for these regions, the state secretary was actually able to direct research policy in the Netherlands towards mission-oriented research as well as towards systems-oriented, higher-level research.

Other health research institutes, organizations, or projects exist outside the sphere of influence of the two ministries mentioned (Querido 1973). However, they are minor within the total picture of health research policy. The Ministry of Foreign Affairs subsidizes the Royal Institute for Tropical Medicine; the Ministry of Defense supports the Medical Biological Laboratory; and private organizations such as the Cancer Fund, the Kidney Foundation, the Heart Foundation, the Foundation for Professional Activities' Survey, and the Fund for Preventive Medicine also support health research within their respective areas. It is interesting to note that the Fund for Preventive Medicine was established by the health insurance agencies themselves. A major part of this fund's efforts, however, go to biomedical research, and only a small part is devoted to health services research.

Health Statistics

The Netherlands has traditionally been a frontrunner in the development of health information and of health resources information systems. Four agencies, which have a close working relationship, have been primarily responsible for developing the existing information systems:

(1) Recognizing the need for up-to-date and usable census data, the Ministry of Economic Affairs set up the Central Bureau of Statistics immediately after the war with a view to developing and coordinating information systems pertaining to all sections of socioeco-

nomic life. In 1950, the first health related statistics were published, including mortality statistics, such as deaths due to congenital malformation, anencephaly and stillbirth; morbidity statistics, such as cardiovascular disease; and hospital statistics indicating the availability of physical hospital resources. This collection of statistics has been developed and expanded over the years to produce real information systems, particularly with respect to hospital statistics. Moreover, the bureau has joined forces with the Foundation for Professional Activities' Survey to report hospital morbidity statistics on a regular basis (Central Bureau of Statistics 1973). In cooperation with the Central Planning Office and the Central Council, the same bureau also reports on health care costs in the Netherlands, although irregularly.

(2) The Medical Inspection Division of the Ministry of Public Health and Environmental Hygiene works closely with the Central Bureau of Statistics and has helped to stress the importance of health information systems ever since the Second World War. Through an act of 1939, this division was made responsible, in part, for manpower deployment in the Netherlands, and it began to collect manpower statistics. In 1966 a coordinating and development-oriented program was worked out to indicate in which directions the Dutch health information systems should develop (De Groot 1972). Different areas for further development were indicated, some of which have already been tackled: noninstitutional morbidity, congenital malformation, psychiatric morbidity and mental handicaps, physical handicaps, and old-age morbidity. In 1972 the Ministry of Public Health and Environmental Hygiene also founded a long-term planning office, which, though not directly oriented towards health information systems, has nevertheless made considerable headway in applying the available health information system to the development of planning models, such as projection models, and simulation models within system elasticity models. This has been done in cooperation with university research institutes and some national institutes, such as the National Hospital Institute. The same ministry, in accordance with the Health Council's advice, is also active in disseminating information and developing information systems concerning variables in health sociology, health education, and so on, and in coordinating national, regional and even locally generated health-related information systems. It is also concerned with the development of managerial guidelines and planning criteria with respect to health delivery and health care institutions.

(3) The National Hospital Institute, founded in 1968, has achieved a prominent position in the development of information systems pertaining to hospital activities. Several data banks have been established and kept up to date. Most importantly, annual surveys are published on hospital costs, hospital activities, and hospital manpower utilization rates. Psychiatric hospitals and nursing homes are usually included in the surveys, as well as acute care hospitals. Moreover, the institute investigates and surveys other areas, such as the current and projected availability of medical specialists in the Netherlands.

(4) The health insurance agencies have only recently started to develop their own health information systems. The heterogeneity of these agencies and their primarily administrative outlook has so far precluded the development of any real information system. However, in 1971 the agencies joined efforts to develop their own information system on the health consumption of their membership—about 70 percent of the Dutch population. The results of this first effort were recently published for 1973 (Landelijk Informatie Systeem Ziekenfondsen 1974) and indicate the potential for uncovering population-based consumption patterns in ambulatory care as well as in institutional care.

It would be unfair to discuss health information systems in the Netherlands without mentioning the work of the Foundation for Professional Activities' Survey (Stichting Medische Registratie 1969). While nearly all health information systems try to indicate patient utilization or resource consumption patterns, this foundation, established in 1963, has developed its own hospital-based information system to relate utilization and resource consumption patterns to population parameters such as morbidity prevalence, and to parameters of the medical care process. The objective of this work is to improve the efficiency, and eventually the effectiveness, of the health care system in general. Although confronted with an enormous task, the foundation has, in its ten-year lifespan, developed a system that reports on some 80 percent of all short-term inpatients; on the basis of this data bank, it has formulated and tested many hypotheses with the object of improving the health care delivery system on a micro as well as a macro level.

The private health insurance companies, working together in the National Consultation Committee for Private Health Insurance Companies, intend to start a health information system (KISZ) similar to that of the sickness funds (LISZ). The LISZ system and the KISZ system and the Foundation for Professional Activities' Survey will probably merge into one overall health information system.

Other information systems are also in operation in the Netherlands, but their development has been irregular, usually related to specific research interests. The issue of computer- or non-computer-based information systems has been shown to be irrelevant. All information systems mentioned use computer technology. The problem is more one of software: most information systems are still data-bank-organized; few are information-system-oriented or have reached the stage of a management information system. Off-line retrieval is still prevalent, though some headway is being made towards the development of on-line retrieval.

In Retrospect

Among the five countries studied, the Netherlands excels through the dominant role of its voluntary institutions in the provision of health care. Through a combination of contributory health insurance and special taxes, and by using regulatory approaches, the government in the Netherlands has consistently sought to raise the required financial resources and to guide the voluntary institutions in building a comprehensive and equitable health care system.

6 | Sweden

The Swedish national health program has evolved spontaneously and gradually (Anderson 1972, p. 80). Choosing the important steps within that evolution proved more difficult than in the other countries, since changes in the Swedish system have occurred in a more incremental way. However, to retain some consistency with the other countries, the introduction of compulsory insurance was selected as the first vantage point for the study. The 1970 Seven Kronor Reform (Navarro 1972), affecting the financing of outpatient care, was selected as a second vantage point. Finally, the 1973 government proposal for Swedish health care in 1980 was chosen as the third vantage point.

A Latecomer in Compulsory Health Insurance

A Supplement to Inpatient Care

Voluntary health insurance in Sweden, as in the other Scandinavian countries, developed from the basic aim of providing "income replacement during periods of illness causing absence from work." At a local level, and especially during the nineteenth century, the workers themselves created "providence societies," or "sickness funds." By the end of the 19th century, Sweden contained a network of these local providence societies, which provided cash benefits or income insurance. Around the same time, the trade unions also started programs to provide cash benefits during sickness. By 1910 there were as many as 2,400 registered societies, with a total of 635,000 members, or nearly 14 percent of the adult population (Lindberg

1949, p. 438). In the same year, the societies, while remaining voluntary, were placed under state supervision and had to register in order to receive certain state subsidies (Riksförsäkringsverket 1975, p. 1). This financial incentive further increased their popularity. Meanwhile, the societies' programs expanded to include benefits in kind, mainly for out-of-hospital physician services.

From 1910 on, compulsory health insurance began to emerge as a public issue, and it eventually became the subject of recurrent official study. In 1919, for instance, a royal commission proposed making health insurance compulsory so that it would cover the whole population and provide for physicians' services and drugs, in addition to disability insurance. Basic features of the act that was passed in 1947 were already advanced in this 1919 study: universal coverage, financing through a combination of contributions and general revenue, copayment by the insured at the time of service, and the allocation of benefits mainly in cash and reimbursement for physician services (Anderson 1972, p. 73).

However, the 1919 study was shelved. Similar abortive government studies followed in 1926 and in 1929. The public hospital network, in which care was almost entirely free at the time of service, because county taxes were meeting the costs, must have minimized the urgency of making health insurance compulsory to some extent. When hospital stays and related costs are covered by general revenue, as was the case at that time, an important incentive to broaden the insurance base is absent. The early Swedish initiatives in direct state provision of health care created a situation in which the role of health insurance was bound to be supplementary and even marginal as a percentage of total health care expenditure.

The development of the Swedish public hospital system was unique; determined by factors dissociating hospital care from the sphere of indigent care, the foundations for a regionalized hospital system were laid much earlier than in other countries. In 1818 the crown imposed a specific per capita tax to finance special hospitals for the care of soldiers afflicted with venereal diseases. Soldiers suffering from these diseases had been returning from the expansionist wars that Sweden had waged until 1809, when the Baltic empire was lost (Anderson 1971, p. 106). The government decided to finance hospitals from the per capita tax for venereal disease even after the disease had lost its epidemic character. In 1862, the national government turned its role of financing general hospitals over to the county

councils, which had been created as a result of an administrative decentralization. This decentralization had been requested by the
farmers, merchants, and tradespeople, who favored a more coordinated approach towards health and social care rather than the traditional, divergent efforts of the parishes.

The county councils employed physicians in their hospitals and
paid them a salary while allowing them to conduct a fee-for-service
practice as well, on or off the hospital premises. Most of the remaining Swedish physicians were salaried by the national government as
district or town medical officers. The role of these district or town
doctors was originally to cope with infectious diseases and to provide
physician services in remote areas. However, they gradually evolved
into community-based practitioners, responsible for general public
health measures, preventive services like school health and maternal
and child health, all under contract to the authorities, and ambulatory care, for which they charged fees. They could furthermore supplement their salary by private practice.

This dominant government role in the provision of hospital care
and ambulatory care was reinforced by the fact that all appointments
of medical doctors in the public health services (hospital positions as
well as district officer positions) had to be approved and funded by
the central health authorities, the precursors of the current National
Board of Health and Welfare. Independent private practice was restricted to the larger towns where there was likely to be a sufficient
critical mass of clientele prepared to pay "higher" fees for ambulatory care. This restriction meant that private practice never handled
more than 25 percent of all ambulatory patient visits a year.

Against this background of a predominantly government provision of hospital and ambulatory care through salaried physicians, the
development of compulsory health insurance focused on income insurance during illness and reimbursement for drugs and for physician fees. Not only the independent private physicians, but also the
government-employed physicians could charge fees for ambulatory
care, whether performed at the hospital outpatient department or at
the medical officer's surgery. The case in favor of compulsory health
insurance was further based on the argument that voluntary insurance seemed to leave out low-income groups and the aged, who
indeed could not afford the insurance premiums. Even for the voluntarily insured, the costs of physician services were poorly covered
and could upset a family budget.

The issue of universal health insurance was revived in 1932 when the Social Democratic party came into power at the height of the economic depression. A royal commission, appointed in 1937, reported on social welfare in general and on health insurance in particular in 1944. Its investigation of health insurance issues centered on ambulatory care by physicians and on drugs. The report considered the expansion of hospital-based outpatient departments and proposed that they offer care to low-income groups entirely free at the time of service. However, it endorsed the principle of contribution through payroll deduction, which was considered psychologically important, since the insured are involved more directly than they are when health care is financed totally from general revenue. Also, a contributory mechanism would be less expensive to run than general revenue financing. Copayments were seen in the same perspective. High value was also placed on the patient's free choice of doctor (Anderson 1972, p. 75). Ultimately, negotiated fee schedules were to be mandatory once the compulsory insurance had started.

Organized medicine, represented by the Swedish Medical Association and strongly influenced by hospital physicians, in particular those in the teaching hospitals, was ambivalent toward the proposed universal health insurance. On the one hand, some physicians opposed compulsory insurance in the fear that physicians would be overworked; on the other hand, younger doctors favored health insurance since the expansion of physician services would give them more work. Presumably, the concern about overwork was stimulated more by a defensive reflex than by hard evidence. This ambivalent position also derived from the ongoing debate on medical manpower needs, in which some contended that too many doctors were being trained, while others predicted a shortage of doctors. Eventually a shortage was confirmed, but in the 1940s, when compulsory health insurance was being hotly disputed, most physicians still believed that an excess of doctors was imminent in Sweden (Charney 1969).

Main Points of the 1947 Sickness Insurance Act

The Sickness Insurance Act was passed by the Riksdag on January 3, 1947. It went into effect, after minor amendments, eight years later, on January 1, 1955. Rosenthal states that "This act did not take effect for a number of years because it was believed that Sweden did not have sufficient hospitals and physicians to meet the demands for service that would arise under the compulsory health insurance program" (Rosenthal 1965, p. 8). However, the eight years that elapsed between enactment and enforcement of the 1947 act were probably due more to the traditional Swedish way of implementing legislation than to a deliberate effort to bring the health resources up to the level necessary to respond to the introduction of compulsory insurance. Basically the act entailed an expansion, in coverage and benefits, of the existing state-subsidized and state-controlled voluntary insurance. It did not affect the established structure of health care delivery. From 1955 onward, only employees were compulsorily insured. The self-employed were excluded. Children under 16 were covered under the name of their parents. The benefits included partial reimbursement for all physician services: 75 percent of the fees were paid according to schedules mutually agreed upon by the medical profession and the Social Insurance Board or county council. Some drugs were fully covered, but most required a copayment. Travel costs above a certain level were also covered. Hospital care benefits were less significant, as most costs were already covered by the county councils' taxes. Dental care benefits were very restricted.

Although the program was based on employer contributions and payroll deductions, it was nevertheless substantially subsidized by the government (Navarro 1972, p. 64). The compulsory sickness insurance program was administered by the existing voluntary funds. In 1959, however, the administration was handed over to a government agency organized at the national, regional (county), and local level. Finally, in 1962, the health insurance program was integrated with the national pension scheme into a single administratively coordinated, comprehensive social insurance scheme (National Insurance Act 1962).

Reactions to the Act

Because the program initially introduced did not involve major changes, it was acceptable to the medical profession, which was consulted extensively, both before the 1947 act and during the eight years needed to iron out administrative problems before its final implementation in 1955. However, during that period another royal commission, headed by Dr. Axel Höjer, director-general of the National Medical Board, reported in 1948 on out-of-hospital physician services. The report, which was unofficial, as it was only endorsed by three of the commission's five members, proposed a salaried service for all doctors, including private practitioners. This proposal threatened not only private practitioners but also the government-appointed physicians who, as hospital doctors or district doctors, were allowed to practice privately to supplement their government salary, and who expected to retain this prerogative under the 1947 Sickness Insurance Act.

Hospital-based doctors, who viewed themselves as independent contractors regardless of their salaried appointment, had bargained very hard to avoid a contractual relationship with the state for the services they would render under the 1947 act. They feared the Höjer proposal not only for its effects on their incomes, but also as a direct threat to the professional freedom they had so far enjoyed. The proposal emphasized an integration of curative and preventive services, for instance, by providing periodic health examinations under one salaried service. The service would be completely free. Opposition by the Swedish Medical Association was fierce, particularly to the salaried service. It argued that the current state of health affairs in Sweden did not warrant the proposed drastic changes, and that other countries with free services (presumably the United Kingdom) should be studied first. The opposition also argued that the preventive health examination required a sounder scientific base, and that it might eventually lead to a need for a substantial increase in resources (Anderson 1972, p. 79).

Although the report was unofficial, it may nevertheless have strained relationships between government and organized medicine, a factor that may have helped to prolong the working out of implementation details of the 1947 act. In general terms, the Höjer proposal launched ideas that were thought sound but unrealistic in an environment that traditionally favored only small, gradual changes. Thus, some of the issues raised by Höjer were ultimately to be resolved much later, in the 1970 reform.

The 1970 Seven Kronor Reform

A Question of Priority

Following the introduction of the 1947 act, a patient visiting a district doctor or a doctor in the hospital's outpatient department paid a fee, sometimes a large one when radiology and laboratory fees were included. Subsequently the patient obtained reimbursement from his insurance fund, but this was limited to three-quarters of an official ceiling, to which most doctors in government employment had to adhere, except for professors in teaching hospitals. Private practice physicians operating entirely outside the system had no limits on their charges, although the insurance funds reimbursed private patients on the same basis as those using the public services, that is, for three-quarters of the fees listed in the official schedules.

The first part of the 1970 reform, which gave its name, the Seven Kronor Reform, to the entire act, introduced a simplified fee system for ambulatory care. In preparing for the reform, a survey and cost analysis was performed to determine the average cost for a visit; including x-ray and laboratory investigation, the cost was determined to be about seventy kronor. The simplification introduced by the 1970 reform charged the patient 10 percent of these costs, or seven kronor, as a flat rate, regardless of the amount of x-ray or laboratory investigation that his visit entailed (Navarro 1972, p. 54).

The second part of the reform, closely linked with the first, affected the method of payment and the income of the state-employed physicians. The existing system, which had permitted state-employed physicians (hospital doctors and district doctors) to charge supplementary fees within official fee schedules to patients for ambulatory care, was replaced by a salary system. At the same time, the rather loose system of working hours was formalized into a specified 45 to 55 hours a week (Werkö 1971, p. 360). Overnight, 90 percent of Sweden's doctors became full-time salaried employees of the state.

Under the previous system, physician incomes had varied widely because of their varying incomes from ambulatory care. Although this variation was somewhat alleviated by the payment of a base salary, the gross incomes of pediatricians and psychiatrists were nevertheless much lower than those of radiologists, ENT specialists, ophthalmologists, pathologists, and other specialists with a high outpatient load. Another problem of the old system was that senior hospital physicians had to decide whether to concentrate on complex inpatient cases when this could result in a loss of outpatient income (Shenkin 1973, p. 555). The Seven Kronor Reform solved this dilemma and also eliminated income differences between specialties by grading salaries by rank rather than by specialty.

Several political issues underlay the enactment of the Seven

Kronor Reform. First, there was inequality in access to outpatient care. In case of illness requiring many tests, x-rays, and procedures, the previous system, it was argued, presented a financial barrier: low-income ambulatory patients hesitated and even refrained from seeking care because of the potentially high fees they might have to advance out-of-pocket, and which were only partly reimbursed later by the insurance funds. A second type of inequality of access was seen in the appointment system for fee-for-service care. The more educated, higher-income groups could cope better with the problems of waiting time, inconvenience, and obtaining access to the senior physicians. Equality has been a constant political objective in Swedish society, particularly under the long-lived (1932–1976) Social Democratic government. In 1968, the Alva Myrdal Report of the Social Democratic party strongly underlined remaining discrepancies in equality in Swedish society, thereby providing specific platform issues for the elections: more equality in education, labor wages, taxes, residential environment, and so forth (*The Alva Myrdal Report* 1971). The same drive for equality not only resulted in the abolition of barriers to outpatient care, but also in equalization of physicians' incomes, both within the medical profession and in relation to comparable professions in the rest of society. Moreover, two corrections were expected to result from this new full-salaried system. First, it was said that the allocation of senior physician time between outpatient care and inpatient care would be better balanced by the abolition of unilateral financial incentives for outpatient care. Second, it was argued that the past discrimination (as reflected in income discrepancies) against psychiatrists, long-term care specialists, primary care physicians, and others now considered important in view of new priorities, would no longer operate. The desire to redirect medical specialization into needed areas was another major issue underlying the Seven Kronor Reform. This concern evolved out of a broader concern about the Swedish hospital-based health care system. By 1970, earlier vague opinions that the Swedish health care system overemphasized hospital and inpatient care had become a firm conviction.

The dominant position of the hospital in Sweden resulted from a number of factors: a long period in which physicians, in short supply, were concentrated in hospitals for reasons of efficiency; the country's extensive area combined with its low population density, which made the deliberate concentration of scarce resources an economic must; the growing prestige and influence of the county councils, who pushed for large, well-equipped hospitals because they offered attractive and prestigious positions to young graduating physicians; the strong emphasis in medical education on specialization and hospital work; and, finally, the growing trend after World War II to consider the hospital as the cornerstone of health care. Thus, by 1967, 64 percent of all Swedish physicians were hospital-based (Anderson 1972, p. 233). In addition to their inpatient work load, these hospital physicians were responsible for about half (1968: 51.8 percent) of all ambulatory patient visits in Sweden, only one-quarter being carried by the district medical officers (1968: 22.5 percent), and one-quarter being carried in private practice (1968: 24.5 percent) (Jonsson 1971, p. 7).

The objective of reducing hospital care by shifting the balance from inpatient to ambulatory care, and by providing ambulatory care in primary care settings closer to the patients' homes and workplaces, was guided by concern for hospital costs. Ambulatory care was believed to be less costly. Further, short-term hospitals could not meet the growing need for long-term care, due to the aging of the population and to the increased numbers of traffic accident victims and other patients suffering from disabling diseases. Therefore, an approach to long-term care involving special institutions and a greater emphasis on rehabilitation seemed necessary (Rexed 1971, p. 201).

Concern over the rising costs of health care in general also underlay the Seven Kronor Reform. During the period 1950–1970, total health care costs in Sweden rose from 1.5 to 18 billion kronor ($0.4 to 4.5 billion), including an annual investment in building and equipment of about 2 billion kronor (Rexed 1975, p. 69). This increase resulted from a population increase of nearly one million, the aging of the population, the concentration of the population in the cities, an increase in the number of doctors and hospital beds, a general rise in prices and salaries, and an extension of medical benefits by health insurance (International Association of Social Security 1972). Taking control of physician's incomes and creating a situation in which the patient could regard outpatient care as a viable alternative to inpatient care constituted two cost-containment mechanisms in one legislative act.

A Dissonant in a Tradition of Consultation

In contrast to the usually gradual process of change favored in Sweden, the Seven Kronor Reform was introduced rather rapidly. Indeed, although the discussions between the government, the county councils, and the medical association were intense, only a relatively short period of time was spent on them, early in 1969. The Swedish Medical Association did consent to the reform, for two reasons: first, anticipating an increase in the number of physicians in the near future, the association preferred to agree on a settlement rather than face more strenuous salary negotiations later; second, the association also preferred to accept the new system of income equalization among physicians because it implied higher income for some, for example, psychiatrists.

Thus, the three months of negotiation centered mainly on defining hospital physician working hours. A basic forty-hour week was finally settled on, which gave the county councils some control over physician time, but which also gave physicians the opportunity to charge for overtime. Indeed, physicians were very well paid for every hour worked beyond forty hours a week, according to a special agreement between the medical association (employees) and the county councils (employers). Before the reform came into effect, the association declared that, "In all the essential aspects it would support the aims of the plan and that the doctors would perform their part loyally." However, the medical profession itself was rather divided, mainly about the central issue, the equalization of professional incomes. Younger doctors clearly favored the salary system. But only the fact that a specific fund would compensate for a number of years those whose income would drop could bring other physicians reluctantly around (Shenkin 1973, p. 555).

One criticism voiced by the medical association was that the reform would strain the specialties in short supply, like radiology or otolaryngology. The association also predicted longer waiting lists for outpatient visits. Subsequently, in 1971, the association conducted a small survey to compare waiting times, patient flow-through times, number of visits, administration rates, and technical investigations in the period before the reform (1968–1969) and in the period after (1970–1971). It found some increase in waiting time, in particular for otolaryngology, radiology, gynecology, and surgery, but the pattern differed greatly from region to region

(Swedish Medical Association 1971). These findings revived, although only temporarily, the argument that the reform should have been more gradual.

The Health Care Plan for 1980

The Need for More Structure and Better Integration

Despite Sweden's early and continuing concern about its health care delivery system, towards the end of the sixties and the beginning of the seventies the lack of coordination among the different components of the system began to require attention (Socialstyrelsen 1973). The existing health care system had evolved historically, rather than being consciously designed. Short-term acute care developed, under the authority of the county councils, into a well-equipped, highly specialized sector, staffed with specialists. Ambulatory care, originally a national responsibility based on the services of district doctors, had started with limited resources and was at first unable to compete successfully with more pressing needs at the national level. Then, ambulatory care began to be provided by hospital-based outpatient departments and private practices. Health insurance stimulated this development.

Psychiatric care was long available only in specialist institutions under national authority. Preventive and public health services were provided by the district doctors, also with state subsidy. In the sixties, the county councils became responsible for the district doctors and psychiatric institutions: from then on, they provided virtually the entire spectrum of health care. Some overlap remained between long-term care and care for the aged, the former a responsibility of the county councils and the latter a responsibility of the primary municipalities. Similarly, the care of alcoholics, which is still officially a national responsibility, remains an ambiguous area. However, although most of the health services were thus brought under the county councils, the services nevertheless continued to function as separate entities, insufficiently coordinated, and with an overemphasis on hospital-based care. Existing legislation tended to preserve this pattern.

The awareness of this lack of coordination in the delivery of health care was accompanied by increasing interest and action in the area of health care planning itself. Up to the mid-sixties, health care planning in Sweden basically involved three parties: the primary municipalities, responsible for social welfare in general, and grouped in the Central Organization of Primary Municipalities; the county councils, responsible for running the health care system, and grouped in the powerful Federation of County Councils; and the National Board of Health and Welfare, the government body in charge of planning health and social services in Sweden. Any health-related policy developed out of intensive discussions among these three parties.

However, from the mid-sixties, several important new government agencies were created to strengthen the coordination necessary for this planning process. As early as 1964, a National Health Planning Council was organized within the Ministry of Health and Social Affairs, under the chairmanship of its undersecretary. This council, a political body consisting of high-powered representatives from all national, regional, and local governmental services concerned with health care, crosses ministerial lines. Its object is to coordinate policy and to determine national priorities for capital investment and manpower in the health sector.

Then, in 1971, the Permanent Committee on Health Planning was established to translate the priorities set by the National Health Planning Council into actual health care plans. Composed partly of politicians, but mostly of representatives from the National Board of Health and Welfare, the Federation of County Councils, the Swedish Medical Association, and the Swedish Nurses Association, this committee's mandate is to supervise the introduction and implementation of a new, totally comprehensive planning system. Its specific role is to coordinate health planning with socio-economic planning, particularly in long-term plans; to develop specific norms and standards as guidelines for manpower and facility planning within the priorities set by the National Health Planning Council; and to encourage the preparation of long-term and medium-term plans (five-, fifteen-, and thirty-year) by the county councils. The permanent committee's national health plan now serves as a frame of reference at the county level for medium-term and long-term planning. At the national level it is also used to approve county council proposals for new investment and manpower. The planning system introduced through the establishment of the permanent committee is comprehensive in two ways. First, at the health care level, sectorial planning, like hospital planning on the basis of bed/population ratios, is replaced by total service planning. All the health and welfare services required for defined and structured population groups are determined. Second, overall health planning must be related to all other county council activities, especially to economic planning.

Preparing for a Long-Term Plan

As the new planning system gradually went into operation, the planners began to recognize that—as well as remedying past ills—their plans would need to take account of likely future problems. Their examination of demographic trends showed that the health care system would have to accommodate certain specific emerging problems. The planners found that, as a result of a constant birth rate, a decreased mortality rate in two age groups (children under five years and women over forty-five), and an annual population increase of 20,000 due to immigration, the total population in Sweden would increase during the period 1970–1980 by half a million. At the same time, the age structure would continue to shift toward an increase in the percentage of people over 65 years: 13.8 percent in 1970, 15.6 percent in 1980, and 16.2 percent in 1990 (Federation of Swedish County Councils 1971, p. 45).

This increase in the age group consuming the most health care is very important, since it determines what should be an adequate level of long-term care within a structured health care system. Further, shifts in the spatial distribution of the population will, by 1980, concentrate some 80 percent of the population in centers of more than 20,000 inhabitants, with 50 percent of the population in centers of more than 100,000 inhabitants; 20 percent of the population will be scattered over 60 percent of the country's total surface. To deal with this spatial distribution, the structure for the primary-care level will have to be flexible; and even at the secondary- and tertiary-care levels, travel distance will remain an important factor. The desire to have high-quality facilities, preferably manned by specialists, near the places where people live and work, will probably become more openly expressed.

Medical care utilization in Sweden clusters around some forty diagnostic groups—for example, hypertension, diabetes, upper respiratory diseases, and urinary tract diseases—that are the prime resource consumers. The planners suggested that priorities would need to be identified, and that skeleton programs—diagnostic and therapeutic procedures, including pharmaceutical treatment, levels of care, and personnel assignment and control procedures—could be worked out to deal with these diagnostic groups. They believe that health policy requires nationally standardized methodology and information dissemination and county council programs and procedures. Finally, any health care structure has to accommodate a range of priorities in health care problems.

Another important step leading to the 1980 Health Care Plan was the "Program of Principles for Open Medical Care," concerning ambulatory care on or off hospital premises, produced in 1969 in the National Board of Health and Welfare (National Board 1969). This program was based on the following assumptions: (1) that many diagnostic and therapeutic activities could be shifted from the inpatient setting to the ambulatory or open setting; (2) that increased cooperation between preventive, curative, and social services was possible in the open care setting; (3) that home care services, patient hostels, rehabilitation services, and physiotherapy could be expanded; and (4) that financial and other obstacles to a free flow between different levels of care could be eliminated. The program stressed the need to provide ambulatory health care in multi-doctor units near the population served. In densely populated areas, the staff of these health centers would include specialists; in sparsely populated areas, only general practitioners would be employed. Public health services, preventive services, family planning, maternal and child health, district nursing services, sick-bay service, and dental care could all be offered at the health centers, together with the advisory and supportive services for home care.

The basic hospital outpatient department would function as the specialist care health center. The central and regional hospitals would be relieved of the responsibility to provide open care for those patients who did not really need the highly qualified diagnostic and therapeutic resources of such very expensive hospitals. The Swedish Planning and Rationalization Institute (SPRI), a research institute established jointly by the Federation of County Councils and the National Board of Health and Welfare in 1968, was invited to work out the board's program of principles for open care, and in 1972 it produced its detailed proposal "on the organization of outpatient care." This served as the cornerstone for the 1980 Health Care Plan, which was proposed in 1973 by the national board (Swedish Planning and Rationalization Institute 1972).

Scope and Content of the 1980 Health Care Plan

The 1980 Health Care Plan is deliberately based on the assumption that no major breakthroughs will occur to change Sweden's morbidity or utilization patterns drastically before 1980. Nevertheless, it is recognized that increased preventive action, changes in lifestyle, changing food habits and smoking habits, and the use of drugs more selectively and for preventive reasons are likely to be important. The plan is further based on a number of implicit criteria: the provision of health care on the basis of need; the principle of free choice of physician, including the possibility of direct access to specialist care; cost-effective preventive care focused on risk groups; integration of health and social care; the provision of care in proximity to the patient's normal habitat and social environment; continuity of care, with providers remaining constant over time, and thus capable of relating to the patient in a personal way and of understanding his social circumstances; and a programmatic approach to the provision of care, within normative criteria for diagnostic and therapeutic interventions, for example, standard or skeleton care plans for given types of morbidity, standard plans for drug treatment, and so forth. The 1980 Health Care Plan proposes three levels of care: primary, secondary, and tertiary.

(1) The primary care level should cover 80 to 85 percent of all ambulatory physician visits, 65 percent of all long-term inpatient (nursing homes) care, all preventive screening, family planning, industrial health, school health, home care, and dental care programs. The population base for units providing this primary care should average 20,000, but the area covered should be adapted to municipal boundaries to permit a high degree of coordination with municipal social services. Primary care should be offered mainly by health centers staffed with generalists whose training has emphasized internal medicine, pediatrics, psychiatry, social medicine and long-term care; specialists in child health, gynecology, and diseases of the locomotor system, given the high prevalence of the latter in Sweden; and psychiatrists. Limited x-ray facilities and laboratory services should be provided, preferably staffed on a rotating basis. A transport and communication system should provide a link with the next care level.

(2) The secondary care level should provide services for an average of 250,000 to 300,000 people. Secondary care is intended mainly for patients suffering short-term, acute illnesses that require

inpatient care, with some 50 percent of the cases requiring life-saving intervention; a limited number of patients needing long-term care; and a limited number of patients needing ambulatory care. Care at the secondary level requires a high degree of specialization and is provided in central hospitals with special technology continuously available or in normal hospitals with a more limited number of specialists and a lesser degree of preparedness. Geographic constraints in Sweden necessitate the use of both types of hospitals. Economic considerations favoring centrally located specialized facilities must be balanced against the requirements of easy access and acceptable travel times to health care facilities.

(3) The tertiary care level requires a population base of 1.0 to 1.5 million people. Tertiary care is limited, with the exception of oncology, to a small number of patients requiring complex, multi-specialist care. Facilities for tertiary care are located physically in secondary-level units and are primarily responsible for development of methods, control of the effectiveness of care given at lower echelons, education, and training. Access to tertiary care is on a strict referral basis.

Special studies were made to determine the distribution of outpatient and inpatient care activities in each medical specialty and at each level of care. This distribution serves as the basis for resource allocation. The structure, as well as the distribution of activities over the three levels, is based on the principle that patients will be referred from the primary care level to the upper levels when inpatient care is required and that they will be referred back to the primary level as soon as they no longer need hospital resources.

The 1980 Health Care Plan is now being implemented. Already some reorientation has proved necessary. Emphasis has shifted from the ten-year planning perspective toward five-year plans in response to the county councils' day-to-day problems and yearly planning and budgeting procedures. In 1976, a change in the economic situation induced a need to contain costs; this reduction in expenditure was made in a way that ensured no level of care would suffer more than the others. At the same time, a third generation of planning guidelines has been published by the National Board of Health and Welfare. Because of deficient information, the traditional budgeting systems approach is in many cases being replaced with "sector programs," based on the evaluation of costs and outcomes in alternative models of health care delivery. Such a sector program, for instance, is now being implemented for maternity care—prepartum and postnatal care—and child care. In the meantime, the Federation of County Councils is promoting the health center concept among its member county councils; some experiments have been initiated.

Human Resources

Physicians

Throughout the nineteenth century, the number of physicians in Sweden remained stationary, while from 1862 onward the supply of hospital beds increased rapidly because of expansion sponsored by the county councils. By 1900, the hospital expansion had begun to require more hospital physicians; by then the issue of physician shortages—a constant in Swedish health care policy ever since—emerged for the first time. As early as 1918, a royal commission was created to investigate a possible shortage (Charney 1969). The 1920 royal commission report acknowledged the shortage, and recommended an output of a hundred doctors per year through maximum utilization of educational facilities. The government in turn proposed an output of 150, and the number of available places for the entrance year in medical school was set at 398 in 1923. A joint committee of the Swedish Medical Association, the Swedish Medical Society, and the Swedish Medical Student Association considered the matter and saw no problem in increasing the production of doctors. In its investigation, this committee took into account the great probability of a compulsory health insurance program, which would increase the demand for physician services.

Both reports, the royal commission report of 1920 and the joint committee report, affected enrollment in preclinical education. The size of the student body rose sharply, and by the 1930s bottlenecks began to develop in the physician education program at clinical level. In 1931, Professor Dahlberg, of Uppsala University, wrote a widely publicized article predicting an oversupply of physicians, on the grounds that temporary physician positions previously occupied by medical students were now being filled increasingly by fully qualified physicians. He also blamed the government for ignoring the 1920 royal commission report by increasing the number of doctors produced to much more than the hundred originally proposed. Dahlberg even suspected the government of a dumping policy, that is, of trying to promote a situation in which new low-salary positions would be created. Dahlberg's views were supported by spokesmen of the medical profession, and even by the director-general of the Swedish Medical Board, Dr. Hellström, who dismissed the higher doctor/population ratios of other countries as "overdoctoring." Others opposed Dahlberg's views. The debate ultimately reached Parliament, where the Conservative party, which opposed the Social Democratic party's educational policies, defended Dahlberg's point of view. The general problem of the overproduction of university graduates became the issue. A new commission was appointed; its 1935 report (the Wichsell-Jerneman report) did not anticipate an overproduction, in view of upcoming compulsory health insurance, and therefore approved the output of 150 physicians a year. Organized medicine strongly objected, however, especially to the imputation that the medical schools were restricting educational capacity in order to protect a professional monopoly. In defense of lower doctor/population ratios, the Swedish Medical Association pointed to the high number of allied health professionals in Sweden, who made fully qualified physicians less necessary. Even the Medical Board (the current National Board of Health and Welfare), headed by Dr. Höjer, pointed out the danger of creating an intellectual proletariat. In 1935, the chancellor for the Royal University, the official in charge of higher education, halved the number of available places in the entrance year from 479 to 203.

The prevailing opinion that Sweden was faced with an overproduction of doctors was also responsible for the policy of refusing permission to practice in Sweden to physicians who escaped from Nazi Germany before World War II. In 1938 a new royal commission looked into medical education because of this question of refugee doctors. The commission reported in 1941 and in 1945. It concluded that the unemployment of young medical graduates was overrated and was due not to overproduction but to organizational defects. However, it acknowledged that a job shortage existed. It claimed that existing medical school admissions would suffice to meet any increasing demand caused by compulsory health insurance. Thus, a status quo in enrollment was proposed (at 185 admissions).

Public discussions flared up again, reinforced by the enactment of the 1947 Sickness Insurance Act. In 1948, yet another royal commission was set up. This committee's work was a turning point in the political discussion of physician needs. The 1948 commission produced a new scheme for medical education, including the expansion of the number of medical admissions to about 300. Concurrently, the National Board—in response to questions from the 1948 commission—reversed its previous position and finally acknowledged a prevailing physician shortage and the need for 7,200 doctors of working age in 1960, rather than the 4,695 that had been proposed by the 1938 commission in 1945.

During the fifties, the medical organizations fought violently against this increase, but the process was underway, and early on the National Board recommended an increase in admissions to 400 per year. Intake in existing faculties (Uppsala, Lund, and Karolinska Institute) doubled, and new medical schools were being planned or going into operation: Göteborg (1954), Umeå (1963), and Linköping (1969). Foreign physicians were being admitted: special agreements were concluded during the fifties with Austria, Yugoslavia, and Bulgaria for this purpose. At present Sweden has some 12–14 percent foreign trained physicians. Swedish students graduating in foreign countries have been accredited. Before 1961 accreditation required a royal decree; since then a more flexible legitimation procedure has been introduced. In 1960, a prognosis report on health and welfare published by a committee headed by Dr. Engel, Chairman of the National Board of Health and Welfare from 1952 to 1967, and an expansion report, published by a committee headed by Dr. Rexed, who himself became chairman of the National Board in 1967, dealt with needed physician increases, the required expansion of the educational system, and the facilities that would be required. Both reports were important, since they not only initiated but also set the course for government action in physician education in Sweden up to the present day. Based upon projections of the National Board, the prognosis report stated the goal of producing 1,000 physicians per year. Up to now, this goal has remained unchallenged.

In 1971–72, the National Board evaluated the 1960 objectives, and this evaluation only confirmed the courses of action taken. As of now, physician resource development is still a high government priority. By 1980 a doctor/population ratio of 1:440 is to be reached. Throughout this long period of concern for medical manpower, a unique health manpower planning process evolved, based on both educational and health care needs and preoccupations. The Swedish educational system offers the government four opportunities to influence physician development:

(1) Admission to medical schools. Admission is restricted, and regulated by the Central Office of the Chancellor of the Universities. Up to 1964, the chancellor was an elected representative of the universities. Now, he is a senior civil servant reporting to the secretary of education.

(2) Medical school development. Two medical schools have existed since the Middle Ages: Uppsala University and Lund University. Karolinska Institute was established in 1877. Göteborg University introduced medical education in 1954. These private universities increasingly received government subsidies and were finally "nationalized" in the late 1950s as a result of general public interest in higher education. In 1963 a new university, including a medical faculty, was inaugurated in Umeä in Northern Sweden. One of its aims was to stimulate economic development in the country's northern regions—an objective that illustrates the interrelationships between economic policy and health manpower development (manpower policy being an instrument of this economic policy). The 1960 Regional Hospital Plan Act had introduced the idea that each of the seven health regions should have its own teaching facility. At the present, five of the regions already have their medical school. One restricted faculty (clinical only) was established at Linköping, in 1969, while another is anticipated at Orebrö.

(3) Faculty appointment. Both the number and nature of faculty positions are subject to government approval.

(4) Curriculum development (Shenkin 1974, p. 347). Physician education is a focal point of Swedish health policy. An initially limited interest in the number of physicians eventually evolved into a concern for the qualitative aspects of physician education. The historic breakthrough concerning educational quality occurred in 1960, when the National Board published its prognosis and expansion reports. Subsequently a physician curriculum reform was introduced in 1969, with an emphasis on behavioral sciences, preventive medicine, social medicine, ambulatory care, and a primary care specialist program, which was further reinforced in 1975.

Three further areas of influence outside education, but within the health care system, offer the central government considerable op-

Figure 1. The medical manpower planning process in Sweden.

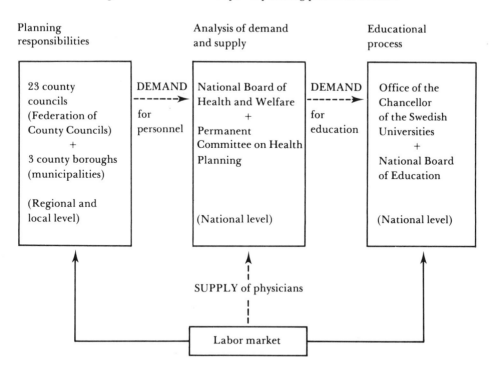

Planning
responsibilities

Analysis of demand
and supply

Educational
process

23 county
councils
(Federation of
County Councils)
+
3 county boroughs
(municipalities)

(Regional and
local level)

DEMAND
for
personnel

National Board of
Health and Welfare
+
Permanent
Committee on Health
Planning

(National level)

DEMAND
for
education

Office of the
Chancellor
of the Swedish
Universities
+
National Board
of Education

(National level)

SUPPLY of physicians

Labor market

portunity to intervene in health manpower planning: (5) accreditation of foreign physicians, (6) number and type of hospital specialist positions, and (7) appointment of district medical officers.

The coordination of action in all seven of these areas is undertaken by the National Board of Health and Welfare and the Ministry of Health and Social Affairs. This coordination has made feasible the integration of physician development within health resources development in general and within the health care plans. In these plans, careful projections are calculated not only for the total number of physicians, but also for specialties and places of activity. The establishment of the Permanent Committee on Health Planning in 1971 facilitated this coordination and integration. Figure 1 demonstrates the current medical manpower planning process in Sweden. The close links in this process between the educational outputs and the needs of the health services system are astonishing. Different factors have facilitated this situation. A first factor is that the purpose of higher education in Sweden is primarily seen as the production of needed numbers of engineers, teachers, doctors, and other professionals rather than as a service to individuals seeking advancement in society (Tomasson 1970). A second factor is the government effort, based upon a traditional consensus policy, to consult all parties involved to solicit their support. The universities, the Scientific Medical Society, the Swedish Medical Association, the county councils, and the university chancellor's office are all represented on the Committee for Postgraduate Training of Physicians, which advises the National Board of Health and Welfare. This committee is only one example of the way Swedish government mechanisms attempt to bring all interested parties together (Rexed 1974, p. 27). Finally, and most important of all, the Swedish government employs the system of medical education, and the type and number of health care workers it produces, in a deliberate strategy designed to bring about changes in the health care delivery system itself. The Swedes have been frontrunners in applying the theory that societal changes should be introduced through a reorientation of the educational system. Reorientation of medical education has been looked upon as probably the most important way to produce the desired shifts towards ambulatory, integrated, and specialized long-term care. This strategy embodies four main principles (Rexed 1974, p. 27):

1. Any reorganization and restructuring of the health delivery system has to be translated into projections of types and numbers of health care workers. The number of training positions required, taking into account attrition due to turnover, retirement, or death, and making allowances for needed expansion, must guide the educational efforts, rather than the educational institutions determining the number of health care workers.

2. The structure of the educational curriculum must suit the changing needs of the health services and should permit the health workers, in particular physicians, to function properly in different settings. A system of life-long education should permit a continuous adjustment to changing needs.

3. All physicians must go through specialist training, including those who will be responsible for primary care. The reorganization of the medical curriculum in 1969 was a reflection of this component of the strategy.

4. New educational programs should be established to meet special new needs.

By virtue of its control over both the supply and demand sides of the equation, the government thus doggedly seeks to match physician production to the defined needs of the country. Progressively more detail and refinement have been achieved in the definition and calculation of needs. The evolving nature of the planning approach also permits projections to be adjusted every two years, to allow for unforeseen developments. Moreover, this planning process has significant spin-offs: an expanding and improving manpower data base and an intricate consultation network.

Other Health Personnel

Development of other health workers has also been very important in Sweden. Dentists, for instance, have received considerable attention. Until 1974, dental care benefits provided by health insurance remained very limited because it was generally felt that, if dental care benefits were more comprehensive, demand would outstrip the supply of dentists. Between 1950 and 1970, the number of dentists increased from 3,430 to 6,720, or by 96 percent. The dentist/population ratio in 1970 stood at 1: 1,191 inhabitants, which is one of the highest ratios in Europe (Socialstyrelsen 1973, p. 71). Dental care benefits were subsequently included under health insurance in 1974, after a deliberate waiting period to let the supply of dentists catch up with the expected increase in demand.

Lower-level health care workers are primarily the concern of the county councils, who are responsible for their educational facilities and wage negotiations. Hospital expansion has created a continuing shortage of nurses. As a result, the nursing profession has become very much integrated into the total health care planning concept: for instance, there is a nurse representative on the Permanent Committee on Health Planning.

The allied health care worker curricula were drastically revised in 1968, under the initiative of the National Board, to bring into focus the qualitative aspects of health manpower development. Higher-level career opportunities were envisioned, to make the professions more attractive. Since 1960, the government has also established new educational programs to meet special or new needs. For example, the training of hospital engineers has been envisioned; and programs have been established for the education of specialists in the interface of medicine with fields like chemistry or psychology (Rexed 1974, p. 27).

Health Care Managers

Until 1970, Sweden offered little formal education in the field of health service administration. In 1940 the School for Social Work and Public Administration in Stockholm offered a three-month course in hospital administration, but it was subsequently abandoned. In 1962 a royal commission recommended a four-year university undergraduate program in hospital administration, in conjunction with the hospital reforms of 1960. But the proposal was rejected because university professors did not consider hospital administration a proper subject for higher education. The Nordic Council, however, acted upon the recommendation, and planned a Scandinavian Health Management Course in Göteborg. Eventually it was launched, in 1968, but was reduced to a one-month program. It was and still is mainly for senior health administrators (Högberg 1971, p. 81). In 1973, formal education in health services administration was started at the University of Lund.

In general, the Swedish health care system seeks its managerial talent among university graduates in law, social sciences, and economics. Physicians, in particular medical directors at institutional and county level, also play an important managerial role. The creation of SPRI (the Swedish Planning and Rationalization Institute) in 1968 was an important step in providing health services research and development in close coordination with the needs of the county councils and the needs of the national health authorities. This institute has effectively increased the sophistication of Swedish health planning and management. It has also stimulated a significant number of persons to prepare gradually for the systems level of resources (see Chapter 1), in three places: at SPRI itself, among the social policy staff of the Ministry of Health, and in the planning division of the National Board of Health and Welfare.

Health Consumers

A voluntary hospital system did not develop in Sweden; therefore there has never been a tradition of public members on hospital boards. Nor are there consumer representatives on the boards of the sickness funds, which have a limited role in Sweden, and which, moreover, were reorganized and centralized in 1962. Since virtually all health care facilities are publicly owned, there are no health care cooperatives. With respect to minority group consumers, Swedish law requires that interpreters be available in each hospital to serve non-Swedish speaking patients. Three aspects of consumer involvement are worth noting: the hospital ombudsman, malpractice procedures, and patients' associations:

The hospital ombudsman. Since the county councils have basic responsibility for the health care system, each county council has an active health services committee; many Swedish politicians believe that a consumer can easily turn to his local county councillor to make complaints or suggestions. Indeed, for the Swedish citizen, the link via the government to hospital or physician is much closer than in other countries. Moreover, there is a national channel to which patients may turn directly: the Medical Responsibility Board—associated with the National Board of Health and Welfare—which deals with disciplinary action for medical personnel, for example, in cases involving malpractice, errors in performance or dereliction in official duties, and the deregistration or reregistration of physicians, nurses, midwives, and physiotherapists. Nevertheless, in the early seventies, a number of politicians, health workers and consumers began to express the belief that an even closer mediation was needed at the local level. Thus, the first patient ombudsman, Miss Birgitta Wistrand, was appointed for the County of Göteborg and Bohus in 1972. The guidelines for this ombudsman program prescribed that it should not constitute a forum for legal petitions, but that cases would be dealt with on a personal basis, as simply as possible. In 1972 the ombudsman dealt with twenty-two cases, and in 1973 with seventy-three. The program proved so successful that five counties now have ombudsmen.

Malpractice. The Federation of County Councils inaugurated a no-fault malpractice insurance scheme in January 1975. Previously, malpractice claims were litigated in adversary proceedings through the courts and took up to eight years to settle. Under the new arrangement, the Federation of County Councils agreed with a consortium of four large insurance companies on a new coverage with a ceiling of 16 million kronor per year (approximately $4,000,000). A patient may approach a claims panel of experts, with or without an attorney. Contingency fees for the attorney are forbidden by Swedish law. If the patient is dissatsfied with the panel's decision, he may turn to an arbitration proceeding in accordance with the National Arbitration Act. During 1975 all simple cases were settled within two months of complaint, and every case within six months. The new act was widely publicized, and is described in the information booklet given to every patient on admission to a hospital.

Patients' associations. Sweden has some seventy such pressure groups, organized to bring about changes not only in the health care system, but in other sectors of society as well. Some deal exclusively with one specific disability, such as the League for the Blind. The largest, the Association of the Handicapped, has 40,000 members, and is open to any one interested in its activities; but the great majority of its members are themselves handicapped. It is organized democratically at the commune, county, and national level. It succeeded in having a law passed in 1968 requiring that all new public buildings give adequate access to the handicapped, and it is now lobbying for a law to insure access for the handicapped to all new publicly supported housing.

Physical Resources

Hospitals

Government action in physical resource development, including hospitals, came early in Sweden, for four main reasons. First, for a long time the Swedes were not wealthy enough that they could afford to build or use private hospitals. In 1870, while most other European countries had already started to industrialize, 82 percent of the Swedish people still made their living in farming and fishing. Second, the size of the country, combined with its low population density, meant that a sufficient critical mass to support general medical practice was difficult to attain, especially in rural areas. Third, the country size and population density also enforced a decentralized form of day-to-day government. Until 1862, when the counties were established, the parish was the traditional administrative unit. Under Lutheran tradition, the parish deaconesses provided simple assistance in a whole range of social and health problems: midwifery, laying out corpses, and so forth. Medical assistance was a specialized luxury, out of place in these communities. Finally, when the national government started its medical officers service in the late eighteenth century, relying on state-run hospitals, a "civil service" medical practice began to be established. Its high esteem and its consequent development minimized the potential market for private medical practice and privately initiated hospitals.

As described previously, Swedish hospitals were initially established and financed by the government in reaction to an epidemic of venereal disease at the beginning of the nineteenth century; and with the local government reform of 1862, responsibility for the hospitals—with some exceptions, such as national university hospitals and mental hospitals—became vested in the newly established county councils. Their power to raise taxes earmarked for hospital care turned them into important hospital developers. Between 1861 and 1904 the county councils nearly doubled the number of hospitals and practically tripled the number of hospital beds. Between 1881 and 1904, therefore, hospital expenditure doubled. As a result "the hospital and the hospital-based specialists became the core of the free health service for the Swedish population, accounting for the still heavy emphasis on institutional services in Sweden and the highest bed-to-population ratio in Western countries up to the present time" (Anderson 1972, p. 43).

This hospital expansion must have been influenced by the medical profession, which rarely met any opposition from the local authorities in determining county health care priorities. Later, as the public began to complain about the high level of taxation due to this hospital expansion, even the ambulatory care model investigated as a cheaper alternative was initially envisaged as an enlarged outpatient department in the existing hospitals. Also, the physician shortage issue was occasionally used to justify centralized health care delivery through big, centrally located hospitals. Moreover, as the need for acute care hospital beds became slowly fulfilled in the mid-fifties, hospital expansion continued, but in other areas, such as care for the chronic sick. (Between 1950 and 1960 the number of beds for the chronic sick doubled. The next decade this number increased by 80 percent [Socialstyrelsen 1974, p. 28].)

By 1967, responsibility for nearly all hospitals had been brought under the sole authority of the county councils, the central government having finally delegated mental hospitals to them. This dominant role of the county councils is reflected in the figures for 1972, when 90 percent of all hospital beds were administered by the county councils or the three county boroughs; 2.8 percent and 0.9

percent, respectively, were administered by central and local government, and 5.6 percent (mainly nursing home beds) were private (Socialstyrelsen 1974, p. 25).

Obviously, this county council drive for hospital expansion and specialization could not go unnoticed by the central government. Over the years, the government took several steps to try to make local initiatives more rational. The first step stemmed from the National Board of Health and Welfare's authority to set guidelines and assure levels of quality, an authority deemed relevant to the building of hospitals. Indeed, any "building investment" over 500,000 kronor ($125,000) had to be approved by the National Board. This requirement allowed the national government to safeguard quality levels throughout the entire hospital system and to introduce many of its concepts into the county council's hospital plans, including timing and size. For this purpose, a special advisory body to the Ministry of Health and Social Affairs was established which had to review all hospital construction plans: the Central Board of Hospital Planning and Equipment. This board also ran a hospital efficiency agency, which served to counterbalance the County Council Federation's Organization Department, which also issued efficiency guidelines. It was through the cooperation of all these agencies, together with the National Board of Health and Welfare, that SPRI was formed in 1968.

A second step that was taken to control local initiatives stemmed from the national government's authority to determine the number and types of medical specialists. County councils were influenced to build certain specific medical departments to the extent envisaged by the National Board of Health and Welfare (Lindgren 1967, p. 46).

Finally, the national government was able to affect physical resource development through its increasingly important, country-wide hospital regionalization planning. The hospital expansion drive during the second half of the nineteenth century led to increased specialization; although this specialization first became apparent in the teaching hospitals, it reached the individual county level soon after (Engel 1968, p. 5). Cooperation among specialists within the hospitals left much to be desired (this was exacerbated by the debate about physician shortage), and between hospitals it hardly existed at all (Lindgren 1967, p. 46). Competition and inefficiency resulted.

From the 1920s onward, some county councils began a county-wide planning effort by developing so-called "central county hospitals," although in an uncoordinated way from county to county (Engel 1971, p. 66). At the beginning of the 1930s a royal commission was appointed to present a "plan of the hospital organization for a county." It was recommended as a guide to the counties, and, like all hospital plans in Sweden, it was not mandatory. Cooperation across county boundaries was called for (Engel 1968, p. 6) and organizational directives became necessary to prevent misplaced investment (Tomasson 1970, p. 10). In 1956 the government appointed Dr. Engel, director-general of the National Board of Health and Welfare, as a one-man royal commission to study the regionalization of health services. In 1960, he recommended a regionalized and hierarchical hospital system, in which three to four counties would cooperate voluntarily to provide highly specialized services at a single regional hospital, which would actually or potentially be a teaching hospital. This regional hospital would serve a population of 1,000,000. Central hospitals would have a population base of 250,000 to 300,000 and district hospitals one of 60,000 to 90,000. Finally, health centers would have to serve populations of 15,000 (Engel 1968, p. 9).

An act of 1960 proposed that the county councils should cooperate in seven hospital regions according to this regionalized hospital system. Collaboration was voluntary. A special standing committee of representatives from all member counties in a region was to act as the coordinating agency. The county that "owned" the regional hospital was to be reimbursed by the other participating counties on a per diem basis (to cover operating expenses and investment costs) (Engel 1971, p. 68). In 1961, a further act delegated to the county councils responsibility for the district doctors and the health centers, to achieve a better integration between medical care inside and outside the hospital (Engel 1968, p. 8). Since then, the regional hospital plan has been the central government's main frame of reference in streamlining hospital resource development.

At the same time, hospital development has been significantly affected by the emerging comprehensive approach to planning the health care system as a whole. For example, the control of hospital investment and manpower allocation are major objectives of the National Health Planning Council established in 1964. The Permanent Committee on Health Planning founded in 1971 is concerned with specific norms and standards for hospital manpower and facility planning, and it encourages the county councils to write up five- and ten-year running projections based on the committee's norms and standards. This committee has also published single running projections, unifying the plans of all county councils, county boroughs, and state hospitals, in 1973, 1974, and 1975. Concerned with plant and personnel allocation and budgetary expenditure, these projections have proved successful in integrating county council initiatives with central government intentions for hospital development. Finally, of course, in the Health Care Plan for 1980, submitted for public discussion by the National Board for Health and Welfare in 1973, the hospital planning effort started at the beginning of the 1960s is developed into a single, comprehensive health care planning effort involving local and national government. Significantly, the emphasis of this planning effort has also shifted from hospitals to the total health care system.

Other Facilities

Health centers, which are still experimental, could provide the necessary facilities for the work of district medical officers. These district medical officers provide primary medical care in Sweden; for a long time, they were rather isolated within the health care system. The posts were often vacant. When, in 1963, the county councils were given responsibility for district medical officers, certain counties started to offer doctors housing, offices, or equipment to attract them to work in their area, while other counties started to experiment with new forms of health care delivery. The health center concept may provide the necessary group practice setting, the paramedical and auxiliary personnel to make the profession attractive, and an opportunity for integration of health and social care at the municipal level. The county councils also run public dental care clinics, educational facilities for health care workers below the university level, and special health care transportation services to cope with the great distances in Sweden.

In 1970, the Swedish Parliament also decided to establish a state-controlled pharmaceutical organization. At present this organization runs almost 3,000 distribution centers, of which approximately 600 are pharmacies. Their activities are coordinated within the health care regional structure.

Information Resources

Health Research

Health research development in Sweden has been influenced by four main factors: (1) the predominance of university institutions in medical research, a factor enhanced by the high social status of university professors; (2) the role of the Medical Research Council, which is the prime source for project-oriented research and development funds; (3) the regionalization of Swedish health care services, by now nearly complete, which embraces all sectors of medical care delivery; and (4) the marginal position of private initiative in health care.

Within this framework, health research policy and the status of health services research in Sweden are changing. There is a publicly debated national concern about research into the expansion and improvement of services. Because of its small population, many people feel that Sweden has to be more alert to research developments than other countries, especially in the case of health research. Of all applicable new medical research findings, Sweden has been estimated to produce only one percent (Lindgren 1973, p. 99); all other research innovations come from other countries. This fact creates the need for alertness and selective judgment of any medical innovations. Only a thorough, research-oriented training of all health workers is believed to generate this capability.

Until recently, the classical areas of biomedical research were emphasized. However, a new need for reorientation has been identified, in particular the translation of available biomedical knowledge "into practical applications in order to obtain a more balanced result, not only from a medical and sociological perspective, but also from the premises of efficiency and resource usefulness" (Federation of Swedish county councils 1971, p. 65). Preventive measures for health and medical care, based upon epidemiological and sociological research about risk groups, have also received more emphasis.

Most health research in Sweden is done within the university departments and is funded by the Ministry of Education through the Central Office of the Chancellor for the Universities. Financial support for medical research activities in the Swedish universities (including about half of the appropriate salaries) amounted to some 150 million kronor ($37.5 million) in 1973 (Rexed 1971, p. 215).

A second important funding source for medical research are grants from the Medical Research Council. The council was created in 1945 to increase medical research opportunities and to improve the allocation of resources for medical research. One objective was to accelerate the evaluation procedure for project proposals, which originally took 16 months, and to create a peer review system. Before the council's creation, proposals were judged first by members of the university faculty, but not necessarily those in the same specialty, and secondly by civil servants unfamiliar with the field. Despite the changes that have been introduced, the council's procedures have recently been criticized and a royal commission has been appointed to look for still better procedures. The appointment of special evaluating committees, which consist of scientists outside the council but are headed by council members, has rendered the distribution of research funds somewhat more equitable. However, the council has not proven itself able to direct medical research policy. Priority areas have hardly been defined, and the council usually acts in response to applications received rather than initiating activity in needed areas of research. This defensive approach clearly favors the already established university departments, which are in a position to formulate more persuasive proposals.

The same attitude, it has been said, has also brought about an undesirable degree of centralization. Those strong research units that, for procedural reasons, are likely to receive more funds, tend to perpetuate their position and to gain an undesirable degree of tenacity and autonomy, even though they remain within the formal university structure. The number of quasi full-time research groups of this type must necessarily be limited. But once initiated, such groups have tended to continue until the group leader retires (Werkö 1973, p. 215). Further, the full-time researchers attracted to these units have been able to develop their own permanent careers up to the professor level, and hence to attain stability.

The research funds allocated by the Medical Research Council increased sharply during its first decade of existence, but recent increases have failed to keep up with inflation. As of now, the council budget is stationary, amounting to 47 million kronor ($12 million) in 1972. This leveling off may be linked to a political desire for more mission-oriented research and for less traditional biomedical research.

In 1960, the lack of a clear-cut government research policy, and the absence of a specific cabinet member responsible for research, led to the creation of a Science Advisory Council chaired by the prime minister and attached to his office. This council has approximately 20 members, well-known scientists, politicians, and others with an interest in science policy; its task is to direct long-term science policy in Sweden. So far, however, the influence of the council in the formulation of governmental science policy is unclear. Either because it has tried to avoid creating political splits between representatives of similar institutions and disciplines, or because of its frame of reference—advisory, with no power to allocate funds—the council somehow has not gained the influence of similar councils in other countries (Germany and France, for example).

A second line of approach towards formulating a new health research policy stems from the county councils and their federation. The responsibilities of the county councils in the administration of the health care facilities have been steadily increasing. Their growing interest in redirecting health research, since they daily confront the problems of improving their health services, is not surprising, for several reasons.

First, the county councils have little control over a considerable amount of the biomedical research being conducted within the university hospitals that they run, even though this activity takes up about 10 percent of the time of the chiefs of services. Although the councils do not want to decrease this research activity, they are not yet convinced that it coincides totally with the interests of the patients. Hence, in the annual congress organized by their federation, the county councils are pushing for greater recognition of the community interests in determining research priorities. Specifically, they emphasize research into the "grey" areas of medicine (common diseases such as rheumatism and psychiatric ailments), and they want to be represented on the bodies allocating research funds.

Second, the county councils bear primary responsibility for health care planning, and therefore are pushing for better health planning methodology and the hard data needed to support it. Also, they want to stress research on medical care delivery and the efficiency of the medical care resources involved.

Third, through their federation, the county councils are also involved in developmental work that requires a certain amount of research support—for example, the development of hospital budgeting systems, experimental health centers, health care workers' educational curricula, and a common county council planning methodology.

A third line of approach towards the formulation of a new health research policy comes from SPRI. SPRI is Sweden's single most important health resource-dedicated research institute. Its purpose is to promote and coordinate the planning and the efficiency of health and welfare services in Sweden, to gather and distribute information, and to establish standard specifications for hospital equipment (Swedish Planning and Rationalization Institute 1974, p. 1). Its unique role—falling between the national government (the Ministry of Health and Social Affairs and the Ministry of Finance) and the local government (the Federation of County Councils)—has been most instrumental in its development of a mission-oriented health research policy. Apart from an important consultant role—hospital building inspection, equipment standardization, hospital organization, and information dissemination, especially in medical technology—SPRI's main contribution to policy development is in translating the results of the general national discussion on the efficiency and effectiveness of health care services into specific operational programs. For example, following national discussion in the late 1960s on the health care cost explosion and what could be done about it, SPRI was a primary contributor to two new programs. The first program dealt with planning. SPRI had been the prime mover in developing planning methodology and defining its information requirements. The resulting planning methodology has been widely and fairly successfully used in the individual county councils' plans. The second program deals with an analysis of the effectiveness of health care delivery. Though this program has proven more difficult to develop, major work towards the development of specific care programs is still going on.

As of 1976, other research areas at SPRI are the development of programs for care of the aged and for primary care. These programs are being developed in pilot experiments in cooperation with the National Board, the Federation of County Councils, and the Federation of Primary Communes (Werkö 1973, p. 207). Sweden also has some other, smaller health research centers with mission-oriented objectives, including the Research and Statistical Department of the Swedish Nurses' Association, established in January 1953, which has been instrumental in reforming nurses' educational curriculum and in the nursing care experiments now being conducted in some hospitals (such as Örebro county hospital); and the Office of Research of the National Social Insurance Board, associated with the Ministry of Health and Social Affairs, which was instrumental in providing the background information necessary to develop the Seven Kronor Reform.

Information Resources

Information and health information systems are well developed in Sweden because of the country's long tradition with national census data. The main strength of the Swedish health information system stems from the country's organization into twenty-five counties and the establishment of a governor's office in each county to act as the central government's representative and to take responsibility, among other things, for a health information census. These censuses have been taken by the Swedish Central Bureau of Statistics since the organization into counties in 1862. By now, this "population administration" is well automated. Elaborate public health statistics have been published annually by the National Board of Health and Social Welfare since 1911. These statistics—collected through the Central Bureau of Statistics or through the Division of Statistics of the Planning Department of the National Board of Health and Welfare—include population census data, vital statistics, economic and administrative data, medical manpower data (covering all health personnel), outpatient care (data for medical officers only), hospital discharge statistics, and hospital administrative and economic data (Tengstam 1975).

Health manpower statistics are rather detailed, because by law every physician, nurse, midwife, and other health care worker must report his address and specialty to the Division of Statistics annually; this division also records vacancies, retirements, and other data every six months. An outpatient care registry in the same division reports annually on the utilization of medical and paramedical personnel in the public sector. Although subjective and imprecise, these data permit an estimate of the number of outpatient visits and their average time. The same division also receives a copy of the annual administrative and economic report produced by each hospital for its county council, which reports the most common hospital statistics. Hospital bed waiting lists—the so-called "care planning" lists—are also centrally collected four times a year. These lists include not only the number of registered and admitted patients for the previous three months, but they also report on admission priority. Other statistics are collected on a voluntary or contractual basis: detailed hospital cost data—investment costs and running costs—are collected by the Federation of County Councils; a hospital activity survey, including diagnosis and therapy, is conducted voluntarily by the Division of Statistics of the National Board and covers more than half of all Swedish hospitals; most professional organizations collect detailed statistics on the nature and activity of their membership; and information on the number and nature of physician visits per insured person is aggregated by the Swedish National Insurance Board.

Special purpose information systems are also being experimented with in Sweden. The most sophisticated is the information system for planning purposes inspired by SPRI's planning methodology. Other special-purpose information systems have also been developed by SPRI or the Federation of County Councils. Most of these involve the standardization of electronic data applications among Swedish hospitals, to make individual hospital statistics comparable—on activity (for example, clinical chemistry activity), on costs (such as detailed bookkeeping data), or on facility lay-out (hospital space utilization). Three recent experimental and developmental information systems deserve some closer attention:

(1) The Karolinska Hospital Computer System (Hall 1974) was the first attempt in Europe to develop a complete integrated hospital information system for patient care, medical education, and clinical research. It was implemented in a 1,000-bed teaching and research hospital with a long-standing reputation. The project was launched and funded by the Ministry of Finance's Agency for Administrative Development, which functions as an efficiency improving agency. This agency made a special agreement with IBM during the project's first phase (1965–1970) for cooperation in developing and testing the system proposed. The project's goals were very ambitious: though many years of developmental work were anticipated, from the start the project aimed at implementing an all-encompassing and fully-automated patient-oriented information system for all patient care activities, including education and research inside and outside the hospital. The basic concept was that, since most physician decisions have to be documented one way or another, and since 50 percent of a hospital's operational costs are due to procedures planned, ordered, and performed by physicians, the core of the computer sys-

tem should be the automated medical record system, to which other subsystems, such as service unit management, administrative and patient scheduling, should be linked. The project gained momentum over the years, and by 1972 had a staff of fifty people. Several subsystems were successfully implemented, for example, an automated multiphasic screening for Stockholm county personnel, some 12,000 individuals a year. However, by 1975 it had become clear that this project would be never ending and would involve increasingly higher marginal costs as new applications were incorporated. In 1976, therefore, the project was discontinued, although the applications developed have been kept in operation.

(2) The Stockholm County Medical Information System, or the Danderyd Project, was launched in 1965 by the Stockholm County Council to cover routine administrative as well as medical and planning functions for the whole county (1.6 million people, 71 hospitals, 20,700 beds) on a real-time basis (Peterson 1975). The system's basic mechanism is an automated population register run by the county council's EDP department: it contains data on the whole population and not just on patients admitted to institutions. Besides all vital individual information, the system also contains so-called critical medical information (such as critical diagnoses), information on inpatient care received, and information on x-ray examinations. Most of these applications are management- or facility-oriented and produce statistics relevant to the short- and long-term planning of the Stockholm County health facilities. Although some of these facilities are already linked up to the system, major problems are arising in the area of ambulatory care. Furthermore, political and financial constraints have prevented completion of the project, and the county council's planners have not yet been able to exploit the full potential of the system for planning purposes.

(3) A project undertaken by Uppsala University Computer Department and the Department of Social Medicine involves the Uppsala area and covers some 22,000 people. Since 1971, all medical contacts in this area have been monitored. Population-based, the system starts very pragmatically—no new hardware has been needed, since there are a number of units within the existing university EDP Department—and has a clear-cut objective: to investigate health care utilization of specific population groups and subgroups. Thus, the project also emphasizes epidemiology. Special attention is paid to those who do not consume health care or consume very little, as well

as to high-risk groups. As a result, new concepts important for health care planning have already been developed: a person factor, which measures an individual's use of the system through the frequency of his health facility contacts, and a societal risk factor, which measures a subgroup's dependency upon health facilities in relation to preventive action. This health information system is still actively in operation, and has been valuable for health care planning in the Uppsala area, especially in linking health care planning with social care planning.

In Retrospect

Back in the last century, when expressions such as "regionalization" and "national health service" had not yet been coined, Sweden initiated developments that produced over the decades a regionalized public health care system based on public hospitals and salaried physicians. Very gradually, and in constant consultation with all parties involved, regional and national authorities have strived to increase the comprehensiveness of the system, to integrate its structure, to optimize its resource mix, and to constantly adjust it to the shifting needs of the population.

II | Government Policies

7 | The Policies

The history of health resources development in the five countries reveals a fascinating picture of how the governments struggled with serious problems and issues that spurred them into action shaped by circumstance, by important events, and often by conflicting forces. At first glance, each country seems to present a unique and unprecedented series of experiences in the unfolding of its national health program. A more thorough examination, however, uncovers a consistent pattern in the five countries: all the governments, in a remarkably similar sequence, made the same set of responses to similar problems, guided by comparable issues and influenced by identical forces and events. By and large, the five countries present a uniform pattern of interlocked and overlapping policies, representing successive shifts in emphasis or consecutive foci of attention with respect to health resources development (Figure 2). The term "policy" refers not only to manifest and explicitly stated government intentions, but also to latent interests and underlying principles that can be inferred, through hindsight, from given courses of action.

The overriding policy at the creation of the national health program or at the introduction of compulsory sickness insurance in each country was to provide access to medical care, primarily by lowering financial barriers to physician services. This objective was not accompanied by a substantial concern for the development of health resources. However, hospitals and hospital development gradually came into the limelight and long remained the dominant concern in the national health program.

The next policy, which was grafted onto the hospital-oriented policy, was a shift of attention to so-called neglected areas such as care

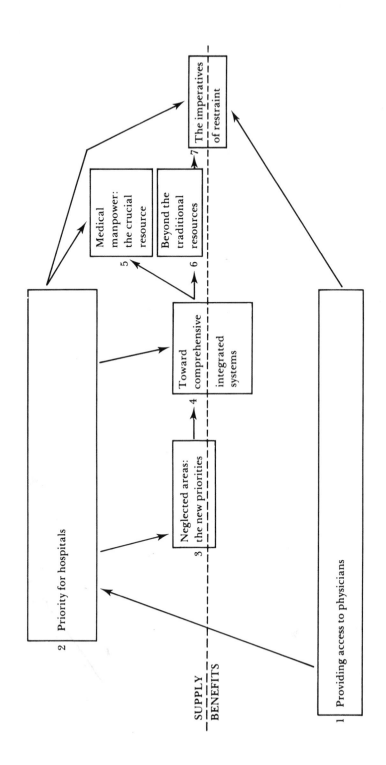

Figure 2. Policies for resources development.

for the aged, the mentally retarded, and the mentally ill. However, these specialized developments added to the fragmentation and the lack of coordination from which the national health program was increasingly suffering, and thus contributed to the emergence of comprehensive and integrated health care plans. The drive towards comprehensiveness and integration gave momentum to the gradual emergence of manpower as the crucial resource. Since then, attention has shifted tentatively from the traditional resources, such as doctors and hospitals, toward managerial and health system resources. Still overshadowed by the hospital orientation, these management-oriented policies have merged with a current policy of restraint and cost-containment in what could be referred to as "resource development in reverse."

A number of political issues have acted as guiding principles for the successive policies. The issues of equity and cost-containment have been important since the very beginning. The "new perspective on health," whereby health is no longer considered to be synonymous with health care is a more recent issue and thus intervened at a much later stage of policy development. Within the myriad of influences that have impinged upon health resources development policies, certain forces have played dominant roles: social upheavals, advances in medicine, organized medicine, academia, the financing of health care, and the different levels of government involved in health care have been instrumental in forging health resources development.

Although they have passed through identical stages in health resources development, the countries have not always moved in phase with one another. Each has progressed at its own rhythm, thereby obtaining opportunities to learn and profit from those further ahead in the sequence at any given moment. Germany's system of sickness insurance acted as a model for a number of other European countries. The reaction of organized medicine to the pattern of policy development also indicates a cross-fertilization on positions and tactics among physicians of different countries. By and large, however, none of the countries systematically evaluated neighboring systems. It is hoped that this study may encourage such evaluations in the future. The analysis that follows considers comparatively the seven main policies that emerged from the examination of the individual countries. The policies are described in chronological sequence, although in reality they overlapped to a great extent.

Providing Access to Physicians

When public health insurance schemes were first introduced in the countries studied, the dominant concern was to make the available medical resources more accessible, particularly physicians, acute inpatient care, and drugs. At the beginning, insurance was far from universal; although it was usually compulsory for the low-income groups of the population, even then it excluded some members of those groups for political reasons (for example, in the Netherlands, "independents"; in Sweden, "employers"; in France, "farm workers"; in the Federal Republic of Germany, "wage earners") or it excluded dependents. From this rather limited base, the coverage was extended to larger population groups in subsequent years, either by expanding the health insurance base or by creating a national health service, as in England and Wales. Depending upon political and financial considerations, the expansion took several decades.

Moreover, at the beginning, the programs offered a rather limited package of benefits, of which physicians' services was the outstanding feature (Table 2). This limited range of benefits in turn offered opportunities for gradual expansion over the years. Thus, at its introduction in Germany, England and Wales, France, and the Netherlands, the health insurance scheme merely provided some of the employed with easier access to the available supply of medical manpower by reimbursing them for the cost of a physician's services. In Sweden, the health insurance program was implemented much later (1955). Although its basic aim was also to improve access to physicians' services, it did so in a country where the total population was already entitled to free inpatient care. This was not the case in the countries that had introduced national health insurance earlier.

Equity in health care was the underlying issue in all the countries. Providing equal access to available health care was the important dimension at the start. A specific goal was to diminish economic inequalities in access to health care, by lowering financial barriers and by reducing dependence on indigent care mechanisms. In the beginning, access was made more equitable only for a very limited number of benefits. The entitlement to care expanded differently in the different countries. In Germany, the package of benefits provided by the health insurance scheme gradually expanded to the point where it is now all-encompassing, but the health care consumer's financial situation still plays an important role in determining the conditions under which care will be rendered. Patients whose income is above a given level have to seek private insurance. In both the compulsory and the private insurance schemes, physicians negotiate tariffs that include higher fees for wealthier patients, thus maintaining the old "sliding scale" principle in remuneration. This sliding scale approach necessarily prolongs the differentiation of patients on the basis of their economic status.

In England and Wales, after three decades of national health insurance, which gave lower income groups access to physician services, the National Health Service, created after World War II, entitled all citizens to access, free at the time of service, to the total range of health services. The French development was somewhat comparable to the German pattern, with physicians continuing to charge fees exceeding the fee schedules negotiated under social insurance.

In the Netherlands, physician services and short-term inpatient care were initially covered for the lower-income groups through compulsory contributory insurance and for the higher-income groups through voluntary insurance, a situation that in practice created two classes of patients. Extended care was paid for personally or through indigent care provisions. In 1967 the principle of equity was applied also to extended care.

Sweden is the country where the principle of economic equality in the access to care has probably been pursued most vigorously of all, within an overall Swedish commitment to equality in general, as well as the particular commitment of the Social Democrats, who were in power from 1932 until 1976. The fact that all hospitals and most doctors have been in government service since early in the development of Sweden's health services has made this high degree of equal access possible.

Social upheavals and wars have played an important role in the development of a policy that aimed at reducing financial barriers to medical care. Bismarck's introduction of compulsory health insurance in Germany in 1883 was greatly influenced by social developments resulting from the 1848 revolution and by his basic strategy of undercutting social unrest within the working class by social legislation. A similar concern in the United Kingdom led to the 1911 enactment of National Health Insurance. Emerging in 1918 from what Lloyd George had called "our bloodstained stagger to victory," the United Kingdom aimed for a return to normal and sought to build upon prewar social developments. Unemployment was the outstanding social problem, and arrangements had to be made so that those unable to pay their health insurance contributions could receive medical attention. The examination of large numbers of conscripts in 1917–18 had shown that, on average, only one-third were fit and healthy, while nearly half were "almost physical wrecks." This heightened an awareness dating from the Boer War and, following the Spanish influenza epidemic of 1918–19, underscored the need for a coordinated approach to health problems.

In France, following World War I, a long legislative process, influenced by the social unrest of the period, finally resulted in the introduction of social insurance in 1930. The Netherlands and Sweden, which both stayed out of World War I, discussed for several decades whether to make their voluntary health insurance programs compulsory. In the Netherlands, the Germans forced the issue in 1941, partly to gain sympathy for National Socialism, partly to harmonize the competing position of German and Dutch industry, by levying social insurance contributions on Dutch employers. This "harmonization" may have represented a kind of precursor for the current calls for the harmonization of social insurance in the countries of the European Economic Community.

In Sweden, the issue of national health insurance was overshadowed for a long time by a controversy over the supply of doctors (which had led neutral Sweden during World War II to forbid refugee physicians from Nazi-occupied countries to practice medicine in Sweden). Thus the national health insurance issue was only resolved there in 1947.

Thus, when the countries studied launched their respective health insurance programs, they chose to provide more equitable access to care by eliminating financial barriers to care. Significantly, the introduction of public health insurance was not accompanied by a substantial concern for improving by increasing or developing the facilities and resources through which health care is provided. The application of the principle of equity expanded only gradually over the decades from the initial concern with financial access to a concern with the development of health care resources to permit equal availability in all regions, and finally to guarantee quality of care to every member of the population. But at the beginning, if resource development was considered at all, the focus was on resources to deal with prominent health problems—for example, the 1911 National Health Insurance Act in the United Kingdom provided for the construction of new tuberculosis sanatoriums because of a concern with tuberculosis.

This emphasis on access to available care resulted from several factors. One factor was that in all five countries health insurance programs were introduced in isolation from the prevailing mechanisms responsible for the development of health resources. These mechanisms were not themselves part of a comprehensive and conscious strategy at the national government level.

Two other factors played a major role in preventing health resources development once the insurance programs had been introduced. First, the medical profession opposed expansion of health insurance programs because it was anxious about a possible loss of income and reluctant to give up any aspect of its independence. The second factor was a concern over costs, an issue that has recently become more visible, but which was in fact important from the very beginning.

A first important issue in the relationship between the medical profession and the health insurance programs was the income ceiling under which an individual became compulsorily insured. For the physicians, these insured patients were a new source of reliable income, but they also constituted a threat to income from private practice. The task of balancing these consequences, and accommodating physicians who wished to derive maximum benefit from the combination of private practice and practice for insurance patients, absorbed substantial energy. A second issue was the question of professional autonomy. In most countries, the medical profession feared that the national health insurance program would interfere with the patient-physician relationship, forcing patients upon physicians, or vice versa. Medical practice would become too dependent upon insurance fund regulations and hence upon the influence of the health insurance agencies.

Germany, as the first country to introduce health insurance, set the pattern that was ultimately to prevail in confrontations between organized medicine and national health insurance programs:

Compulsory health insurance was limited to individuals under a given income ceiling.

Patients were given freedom to choose a physician.

The medical profession was given diagnostic and therapeutic freedom, including control over location, conditions, and tools of practice.

Adequate remuneration was ensured for physicians.

Adequate professional representation was ensured in the operation of the insurance programs.

Throughout the evolution of national health programs, the medical profession everywhere strove to guarantee its members a high degree of freedom. To achieve such freedom, the profession resorted to several stratagems, which it has employed consistently until the present.

In the first place, the profession's views about medical independence were highly publicized, constantly repeated and reinforced, until they became vaguely accepted as unwritten law for all parties involved. In a number of cases, particular freedoms were actually written into legislation. The 1911 National Health Insurance Act in England and Wales included specific statements on patient choice and remuneration methods, to meet the profession's requirements. A deadlock in the negotiations over the 1946 National Health Service Act was broken only by an agreement between the medical profession and Aneurin Bevan, the minister of health, which excluded a salaried service for physicians. Bevan lived up to his promise with the 1949 Amending Act, which actually prohibits a salaried service.

In the second place, in every country the medical profession, first among the health professionals, strengthened its national association, and in some countries formed union-type organizations—occasionally rather militant, like the Hartmannbund in the Federal Republic of Germany and the Syndicats Médicaux in France—to defend its membership's interests in confrontation with either the government or the social insurance funds. Third, the medical profession consistently sought to be fully represented in the administrative structures set up to manage the national health program. This was one of the important issues during almost fifty years of confrontation in Germany between the physicians and the sickness funds, which ended in July 1931 with the physicians' victory. Likewise, in England and Wales, the medical profession prevailed against local administration of the 1911 National Health Insurance Act, just as it later achieved its objective that the hospitals in the National Health Service would not be run by the local authorities, but by regional hospital boards in which professional interest could be effectively represented.

Fourth, physicians attempted to ensure that certain aspects of the programs be placed under peer control, in order to guarantee the compliance and goodwill of the medical corps. Examples include fee schedules (France), disciplinary action related to utilization review (Federal Republic of Germany), distinction awards to supplement physician income (England and Wales), spatial distribution of medical manpower (the Netherlands), and hospital management (Sweden). A fifth mechanism was an effort to ensure that any new developments in the health care area—for example, the emergence of allied health professionals, the development of health related information systems, developmental work on new modes of care delivery, or managerial improvements—always center around and concede the pivotal role of the medical profession as the principal source of health competence.

A last but very important mechanism was to ensure that governments permit doctors to combine practice in the national health program with private practice, or to practice within the national health program under special arrangements.

There is a remarkable universality in the way these mechanisms designed to ensure professional autonomy and medical dominance of the national health program have been employed by the medical profession throughout the world. In the USSR, where the total health care system is managed and controlled by physicians (in principle, by practicing physicians, from the federal minister of health, currently heart-surgeon Academician Petrowsky, down to the baseline polyclinic director), the profession pursues the same autonomy and dominance. In 1968, the late Dr. Bogatyriev, at that time director of the Moscow-based Semashko Institute of Social Hygiene and Public Health Organization, made this revealing off-hand remark to Jan Blanpain: "We try to limit the involvement of economists in our health care system to prevent them from shifting our resources to other sectors of our economy." Blanpain, who at the time of that remark was visiting the USSR as a consultant for a World Health Organization traveling seminar on national health planning, was also permitted by Professor Popov, head of the federal health planning division, to state in his description of the Soviet health care system that, within limits, a private system was tolerated within the main system. Another example of the international influence of physician chauvinism occurred when Blanpain happened to be in the Arabic peninsula on a WHO-UNDP planning assignment in 1970. The first USSR-trained Yemeni *feldschers,* young physician-substitutes, had just returned to their home land. During an audience with the Minister of Health, Blanpain noted with astonishment how these young allied health professionals, in the absence of physicians, were pressing for autonomy within their national health service.

This universality in the behavior of organized medicine vis-à-vis national health programs results to a great extent from exchanges with other countries, as exemplified by the Yemeni episode. Educational exchanges and numerous opportunities for contact through international professional gatherings have provided the leaders of organized medicine in each country with ample opportunities to copy and employ the mechanisms that emerged in Germany in the confrontation with the sickness funds. In general, this complex of mechanisms has created such resistance to change, especially when important reforms are at hand, that open conflict has occasionally resulted—for example, the doctor's strike in Germany in 1909.

Occasionally, too, the leadership of the medical profession has been overconfident and overplayed its hand. For example, in the United Kingdom, Lloyd George, while introducing the National Health Insurance Act in 1911, and Aneurin Bevan, while bargaining with the medical profession for the introduction of the National Health Service in 1946, both astutely appraised the political mood at the grassroots level, which supported the government's initiatives, and ignored the profession's representatives.

As mentioned earlier, cost-containment, although of recent coinage in health care jargon, was an issue at the very beginning of national health programs and was the second major factor preventing health resource development at that time. In principle several approaches to cost-containment are possible: limits on benefits, cost-sharing, utilization control, and control of the supply of health services (which implies minimal development of health resources). Because of the emphasis on economic equality in access to health services, benefit limits and cost-sharing mechanisms, which were used at the start, tended to be gradually reduced, and eventually they were virtually abolished in Sweden and the United Kingdom. In the Federal Republic of Germany, the Netherlands, and, in particular, France, where the medical profession has consistently insisted on cost-sharing to reduce the demand for health care, some, though limited, forms of cost-sharing remain. However, even in these countries, serious doubts exist whether cost-sharing measures genuinely constrain costs.

Utilization control and control of the supply of health resources became important issues at a later stage, although Germany very early established a tradition of utilization control for community-based physicians; the procedures used were similar to those employed in the United States since 1972 through the Professional Standards Review Organizations. One result of the 1931 German agreement between the medical profession and the sickness funds was that physicians' activities would be monitored; in return, physicians would be involved in the administration of appointments to insurance practice, and the relationship between physicians and the sickness funds would be legally protected. The utilization control procedure in Germany involved the following steps:

1. The physicians treating sickness fund patients were organized into sickness funds affiliated physician groups.
2. These physician groups designated peer review committees with the specific task of supervising medical utilization within their specific sickness fund.
3. The sickness funds collected all the necessary statistics for the peer review committees.

However, the monitoring system developed by each fund only provided a record of the contacts between a single physician and a single patient. The system did not indicate whether a single patient consulted different physicians, nor did it monitor the total number of patients seen by a single physician. Average rates of medical activity were established for each specialty, and those physicians showing significant deviation from these national averages were identified. But there was little concern about the steadily rising national averages, and action against offenders was limited (remuneration for excessive utilization was reduced). In the other countries, no such early use of utilization control occurred.

Priority for Hospitals

The two decades (1945–1965) following World War II were characterized by a predominance of hospital affairs and hospital development, in particular of short-term acute hospitals. This preoccupation with hospitals as basic resources resulted from a combination of factors that varied in force from country to country. World War II itself directly and indirectly contributed to the priority position of hospitals. A crucial role was played by a cluster of important advances in hospital-based medicine, resulting in policy development being driven by medical technology. Postwar reconstruction also had a significant effect on the development of hospitals. Increased demand for inpatient care, partly resulting in some countries from easier access through health insurance, played an important role. Finally, the powerful position of the hospital-based medical profession and of hospital-related academics, such as those in medical schools and research centers, helped to focus attention on hospitals. Hospitals themselves attracted this attention, particularly from the government, because being capital and labor-intensive and limited in number, they were more visible and easier to identify within a huge but splintered community of health care providers. This combination of forces coalesced to create a hospital-centered vision of the health care system.

An initial consequence of World War II was an even greater awareness of the need for equity in both access to and provision of health care. In preparing for the war, the United Kingdom especially was greatly concerned about the vulnerability of its population and its concentrated industrial capacity, particularly during air raids. This concern, which gave impetus to plans for regionalization of industry, also led, in 1938, to the creation of the Emergency Medical Service, mandated to cope with war casualties. The creation of the Emergency Medical Service led to a renewed interest in the population's health status and ways to improve it and contributed, more than is generally realized outside the United Kingdom, to the ultimate creation of a National Health Service in 1946.

The survey of British provincial hospitals conducted during the planning of the Emergency Medical Service showed that the hospital situation was even worse than suspected, lending force to the conviction that a national remedy was long overdue. Treasury financial support of medical specialists and voluntary hospitals for their services in the Emergency Medical Service provided leverage for the later nationalization of all hospitals. The medical specialists learned that direct access to Treasury money was not despicable, and the voluntary hospitals simply could no longer forego the income from government subsidies.

After three decades of health insurance as the means to give lower-income groups access to physician services, the National Health Service created after World War II provided all citizens with access, free at the time of service, to the total range of health services, including hospital care. The enormous sacrifices demanded from the total population during the war could be compensated only if existing social inequalities were rectified.

Besides reviving the political issue of equity, World War II (and the Spanish Civil War just preceding it) had a significant effect on the development of medical technology, which in turn contributed to the postwar emphasis on hospitals. Henry Sigerist is probably the most illustrious medical historian to have drawn attention to war as a macabre challenge and stimulus to medical innovation. Ironically, war provides opportunities for experimentation on a scale that is normally unacceptable in times of peace (Sigerist 1960, p. 340). From 1936 to 1939, the Spanish Civil War provided the first opportunity to use blood transfusion on a massive scale for both military and civilian casualties, and to improve donor organization, conservation techniques, and transport procedures. All the armies involved in World War II paid great attention to blood transfusion services, and by the end of that war civilian donor networks and blood banks were firmly established (Verdoorn 1972, p. 647). Similarly, the gradual introduction of postoperative recovery rooms in civilian hospitals after World War II was based on the positive experience with such units in military medicine.

However, the most dramatic example of war-related medical innovation was the discovery of penicillin. In 1929, the English bacteriologist Alexander Fleming stumbled by accident—he had been negligent in his inoculation technique and had infected his bacterial cultures with a fungus—on a product emitted by the fungus that had the power to kill bacteria. He called this substance penicillin (Fleming 1929, p. 10). Unknown to him at that time, as he admitted later when receiving the Nobel Prize for this discovery, a French military doctor, Ernest Duchesne, had already made the discovery in 1897. Duchesne's discovery had not been accidental, but was the result of a scientific investigation to prove an hypothesis that had been advanced by Pasteur and his followers about antagonism between microorganisms (Duchesne 1897). It took World War II, however, to marshal the needed massive research and development resources, permitting Florey and Chain in 1942 to bring a discovery nearly half a century old to the stage of patient application (Verdoorn 1972).

Immediately following the war, the innovations and discoveries

that had been made were subjected to a period of explosive development. Sulfonamides and antibiotics, permitting infection to be successfully combated, became widely available. Important advances
were made in anesthetics: respirators were introduced and anesthe-
siology emerged as a separate specialty. Increased understanding of
the pathophysiology of shock led to improved treatment. As mentioned above, organized blood banks became a standard feature, and
postoperative recovery-rooms were introduced as precursors to intensive care units. The uses of x-ray apparatus were expanded and
diversified. Blood chemistry, electro cardiography, and electroen-
cephalography provided potent diagnostic tools. Surgical and ortho-
pedic techniques were improved and became more invasive.

The increased use of motorized ambulance services reduced the
time necessary for life-saving interventions. The expansion of
emergency departments in hospitals reduced this time even further.
Ultimately, the introduction of a general telephone number for
emergencies, combined with these developments, not only helped to
create a hospital-oriented reflex within the public at large, but also
provided the dramatic events that lifted hospitals from their image
of the past. Previously tainted with the stigma of desperation, hospitals entered a new era based on the triumphs of science and life-
saving miracles, and promising more to come.

As well as the dramatic expansion of war-provoked technological
innovation, the postwar period saw most countries embarking on extensive programs of reconstruction, which often included hospitals.
France, England and Wales, the Netherlands, and especially Germany came out of World War II with many hospitals damaged, destroyed, or hopelessly out-of-date because of a prolonged lack of
capital investment. Thus, an impressive hospital reconstruction program was launched, its timing in the different countries depending
on economic priorities. France, for instance, gave priority to the
reconstruction of factories, railroads, and bridges. The impetus to
invest in hospitals ultimately proved very difficult to stop, even after
overcapacity was acknowledged. England and Wales did not embark
on a hospital building spree after the war, because, although the war
had left the hospitals extensively damaged or destroyed, the country
was also short of capital, lacking in building materials, confronted
with an unfavorable trade balance, losing a colonial empire, and
under pressure to enter into an expensive rearmament program in
response to the Cold War (Lindsey 1962, p. IX). Hospital recon-

struction and expansion were delayed again and again. Direct budgetary allocations from the Treasury for capital investment, and the requirement that unspent allocations be returned to the Exchequer at the end of the fiscal year, together with central planning of hospital development, resulted in a tendency to let the general economic welfare of the nation override the need of the National Health Service for hospital improvement and expansion (Eckstein 1958, p. 274).

Confronted with this predicament, the central planning agencies in England and Wales responded more quickly than those in other countries to the messages emanating from health services researchers like Robert Logan, Gordon Forsyth, and others, who predicted that there might be less need for short-term inpatient accommodation than was generally believed (Forsyth and Logan 1960). More than ten years before the other countries, England and Wales had a government policy of reducing the number of acute short-term general hospital beds. The 1962 Hospital Plan was based on 3.3 beds per 1,000 population, already much lower than the 4.5 to 5.5 beds used as norm elsewhere. This policy was partly caused by budgetary difficulties and partly based on scientific investigation into the need and demand for inpatient care. In any event, among European countries, demand and need studies were pioneered in the British Isles, and were undertaken much earlier there than in France, Germany, or the Netherlands, reflecting the tendency of health services research to respond to the problems confronting the health care system (Blanpain and Delesie 1976). Although Sweden stayed out of World War II, it continued to invest steadily in its public hospital system, which ironically had been established in response to the last of the wars that Sweden had waged. When Swedish farmhands had returned in 1815 from military service on the European continent, many had been afflicted by venereal disease. From 1818, a special tax was levied to finance the state program against venereal disease, and this tax went to support "cure-houses" all over Sweden. The Swedish hospital system was thus established and was steadily developed by the county councils from 1862 (Anderson 1972, p. 40). Therefore, Sweden had a headstart in hospital development, and after World War II its high-rise, compact, and technically advanced hospitals provided a model for the postwar hospital building boom throughout the rest of Europe.

Policies providing easy access to hospitals (inherent in the introduction of national health insurance) also enhanced the position of the hospital as a priority resource. Demand for inpatient care rose, resulting in increased hospital admission rates. In France, Germany, and the Netherlands, access was increased by including inpatient care in the benefit package offered by the social insurance system. In France, the renewal of public hospitals was delayed. The prolonged, dilapidated state of a good number of these public hospitals, together with a lingering atmosphere of indigent care, was partly responsible for the development of many small private hospitals, many of them profit-making. Bridgman estimates that in 1968 the number of surgical and maternity cases treated in private hospitals surpassed the caseload of public hospitals, and that, of a total of 300,000 beds, one-third were in private hospitals, half of which operated on a for-profit basis. These private hospitals were eligible for reimbursement by social insurance for services performed, if they complied with technical standards issued by the Ministry of Health (Bridgman 1971, p. 340). Eventually, the renewal and expansion of the French public hospital system got underway, supported by a special health resources development fund. A percentage of the social insurance budget allocated for capital investment financed this fund. For some time, the government in France was ambivalent toward private hospitals. On the one hand, it was admitted that they provided a substantial part of the services; but, on the other hand, there was a desire to replace them gradually with larger, more comprehensive public facilities. Officially, the private hospitals were ignored as much as possible: for example, they rarely showed up in official statistics.

Characteristic of this situation were the French attitudes expressed in Rome in 1966 when hospital association representatives from the six member-countries of the European Economic Community met for the first time to establish what has since become a consultative platform of European Hospital Associations. The French delegation, composed only of representatives of the public hospitals, became very upset at the composition of the delegations of other countries. They took offense at the presence of Blanpain and Prims, representing the Belgian voluntary hospitals, and Monsignor Mühlenbrock, representing the German Caritas hospitals. At one point they refused heatedly to discuss the issue of voluntary hospitals at all, not acknowledging that these hospitals represented 75 percent of the beds in the Netherlands and 45 percent in Belgium, for example, and thereby also overlooking the realities of the private sector in their own country. More recently, the tide has turned in France, and the prevailing philosophy today is to acknowledge the role of private hospitals. They are seen as partners of the public hospitals, with whom they constitute a public service, and both are eligible for public support.

The Netherlands, within its tradition of nonprofit voluntary hospitals, underwent important hospital development as a result of increased demand made possible through social insurance. Loans with or without state-guarantee financed the capital investment. Interest on loans, within reasonable limits, and depreciation costs could be included in the health insurance reimbursement rates. Thus, social insurance supplied important financing for hospital construction. In the Federal Republic of Germany, social insurance has not been used to reimburse capital investment costs, and its role has been limited to matching operational costs of services rendered. The 1972 German Hospital Finance Act, which provides general revenue subsidies for capital investment, tied to compliance with the national hospital planning, thus came to the rescue of the German hospitals.

Within organized medicine, hospital development was promoted by the academic sector of the medical profession, rather than by the practicing physicians who had forged the issues and waged the controversies over compulsory health insurance in the first half of the twentieth century. While organizations such as the British Medical Association in Britain or the Hartmannbund in Germany, representing the rank and file general practitioners, were prominent at that time, the professors, the top clinicians, and the emerging group of basic scientists showed a certain aloofness, although they were prepared if necessary to serve as mediators—for example, in Germany in 1913 when negotiations broke down and the faculty of the Berlin Medical School acted to prevent a national doctors' strike. Once in a while, in fact, an academic voice even spoke up in support of a national insurance plan. Dr. Moore, professor of biochemistry at the University of Liverpool, did so during the preliminaries of the 1911 National Health Insurance Act, to the dismay of the profession at large (Brand 1965, p. 217).

During the period 1945–1965, however, the academic establishment played an important role in strengthening the position of the hospital and in developing a hospital-oriented policy. Teaching hospitals, medical schools, royal colleges, academies of medicine, and medical research councils were among the institutions through which the academics influenced this policy. Their influence extended along several lines. The position and power of teaching hospitals became substantially greater. Emerging theories about medical education, following the Flexnerian model, sought to forge a closer relationship between the clinical sciences in the medical curriculum and the underlying natural sciences. Integration—the integration of advanced patient care (both inpatient and ambulatory care) with clinical research and fundamental research, and with undergraduate, postgraduate, and continuing education—became an explicit objective that encouraged teaching hospitals to expand into large, complex academic health sciences centers.

This development occurred in all five countries, but was particularly noticeable in France, where special legislation in 1958 resulted in the creation of twenty-three academic health sciences centers. In these centers, existing or future teaching hospitals and medical schools were ordered to merge in order to provide patient care, research, and education on a cooperative basis. Concern within French academic circles about the relatively slow progress of clinical medicine in France, compared with the United States, was an important underlying factor. In particular, the fact that France had had no Nobel Prize in medicine since Charles Nicolle received the award in 1928 for his discovery of typhus fever made French academics acutely aware of the existing gap between research in the basic sciences and the clinical domain of patient care (Steudler 1974, p. 83). In order to facilitate this link between basic and clinical sciences, the 1958 decree in France aimed at strengthening the medical staffing of the newly established academic health sciences centers, by introducing salaried full-time staff and dual appointments in a center's hospital and medical school components.

In the Netherlands, the Federal Republic of Germany, and to a lesser degree in Sweden, ambitious building projects for large academic health sciences centers were also launched in the mid-fifties (Blanpain 1968). In England and Wales, when the National Health Service was created, the medical teaching centers asserted their independence by having themselves administered by boards of governors directly under the control of the Ministry of Health, rather than coming under the authority of a regional hospital board. The Royal Medical Colleges, which include most university medical professors, thus ensured that teaching hospitals would have differential treatment and the access to superior resources without which "medicine is bound to decline all over the nation" (Chester 1969, p. 31).

This strengthening of the role and position of teaching medical centers everywhere as the nearly exclusive environment for medical education had a very great influence on the attitudes of medical personnel, orienting them toward the natural sciences and hospital-based medicine. It also provided leverage for the rush to specialization, and for the improved financial rewards, resources, and government attention accorded to hospital-based medicine. A second way in which the academic establishment has influenced hospital development is through constantly advising those preparing national health programs. Whether the national health program is a state service, providing health care directly, as in England and Wales, or a health insurance program, financing health care by regulated independent providers, as in the Netherlands, planning of these systems relies heavily on consultation with advisory bodies and delegated decision making. Elitism—the conviction that health care is the responsibility of scientists—has led to a high concentration of professors and scientists in the numerous councils and committees concerned with national health programs and related activities such as education, research, and management. The hospital-oriented viewpoints prevalent at medical schools and research institutions thus tend to prevail in the advisory bodies as well. Some of the weak points of national health programs, such as overemphasis on sickness instead of health, and neglect of preventive care and health education, reflect similar weak points in the academic perspective.

Thus, all the forces described so far—the war, medical technology, improved access to medical care, the orientation of the medical academics—contributed to the view that the hospital, in particular the general hospital, should ultimately become the organizational if not the physical base from which total and comprehensive care would be offered to the surrounding community. Consequently proposals were made to unify previously separate services on the same hospital site, such as services for the mentally ill, chronically ill, and acutely ill. A strengthened link with general practitioners (preferably also involved in the hospitals) was also suggested. A typical example of such hospital-centered health care was the model presented for Birmingham at a Nuffield Provincial Hospitals Trust Symposium in 1963 (McKeown 1965). Similar proposals were considered in the other countries. Ultimately, however, the hospital-centered model of the health care system was to recede as shifts in policy took place.

In directing hospital development, the different countries moved toward a regional planning process at varying rates. England and Wales, Sweden, and France, adopted this approach much earlier than the Netherlands or the Federal Republic of Germany, establishing structured, hierarchical, three-level hospital systems within defined geographical areas, where the needs of given and expected population groups were to be met by adequate hospital facilities. In fact, only in this decade have the Netherlands and Germany started to consider regional planning. Interestingly, Germany, the last country to embark on regional planning, is also the only one where the hierarchization of hospitals seems to have met explicit opposition on the basis that it might lead to discrimination in quality at the different levels of hospital care.

Neglected Areas: The New Priorities

Although the major emphasis after the war was on the creation of an extensive specialized hospital system providing acute inpatient care, toward the end of the fifties and beginning of the sixties, the needs of different patient groups began to become more prominent. A new awareness of the problems of the aged and the mentally ill led initially to attempts to accommodate them in specialized institutions. However, in some cases this approach was soon perceived to be little more than a stopgap. Ultimately, the new priorities for these patient groups led to the move for more comprehensive and integrated health care systems.

The problems of caring for the aged were exacerbated as their percentage of the total population began to increase, presenting a growing demand for care. Except for the Netherlands, where in 1965 roughly 10 percent of the population was 65 years and older, the other countries had in 1965 reached 12 percent, with clear indications that this proportion would increase further. A trend toward more nuclear family structures and cramped housing conditions, in particular in the Netherlands, and the increasing tendency for married women to seek work outside the home were factors contributing to the demand for facilities for the aged and for mentally retarded children. Not only were these patient groups now becoming more prominent, but the means proposed for caring for them had changed. Specialized institutions were increasingly seen as the places to care for the chronically sick, in particular the elderly, and for the feeble-minded. The general hospitals were considered too expensive to meet this pressing demand, and the chronically ill patient in an acute short-term hospital was thought to be occupying a bed too costly for his condition. The first solution attempted was to create separate extended-care institutions for these patients. However, sufficient facilities of an adequate standard were lacking. Thus, it was gradually realized that extended care would require new modes of provision and new sources of financing. Dr. E. Michel Bluestone, who at Montefiore Hospital in the Bronx in New York City had in 1947 pioneered hospital-based home care (Klarman 1963, p. 60) as an answer to some of the problems of the aged, and who saw his formula spread to many parts of the United States, crusaded in Europe for hospital-based home care. His appearance at the 1958 International Hospital Federation Congress in Brussels received great attention, but apart from a few experiments in Belgium and France, the transfer of the chronically ill from general hospitals into separate, preferably specialized, institutions went on, driven partly by cost-saving expectations.

Other important developments took place in the field of mental health. The advent of chemotherapy in psychiatric care complemented an increased awareness of the deplorable conditions suffered by a great number of mental patients. The potent drugs provided an important technological stimulus towards expansion and modernization of mental health facilities and programs. The solutions for the problems of these so-called neglected areas were at first largely quantitative: more physical resources and an increase in qualified personnel. Furthermore, each country responded to the problems differently. Slowly, however, the solutions began to move toward alternatives to institutionalized care.

In England and Wales, in 1956, the Guillebaud Committee, which had been established to review the cost of the National Health Service, stepped outside its mandate to recommended provisions for the aged (Watkin 1975, p. 150). In 1962 the Medical Services Review Committee took the same position, and that year a first hospital plan was designed to reorient goals. Eventually the government followed the trend in its 1968 and 1970 green papers, and a reorganization of the National Health Service was implemented in 1973 with a view to the reformulated objectives.

Meanwhile, the 1959 Mental Health Act, following the recommendations of the Percy Commission on the Law relating to Mental Illness and Mental Deficiency, made sweeping reforms. It repealed fifteen acts completely and thirty-seven acts in part. It brought all categories of mental disorder—the mentally ill, psychopaths, the severely subnormal and subnormal—under the same legislation and made sufferers uniformly entitled to comprehensive care. Further, while emphasizing community care, it outlined the distinct roles of the hospital service and the local authorities (Watkin 1975, p. 392). Local authority mental health services were not provided through specific grants, as the Percy Commission had recommended, but as part of a general grant. The minister of health was empowered to ensure that the local authorities developed a full range of community services for those mentally handicapped who did not need inpatient care but required residential training centers, occupational centers, or social centers.

In Sweden, the county councils, which had been responsible for general hospitals since 1862, were in 1961 given responsibility for district doctor's service and in 1967 for mental hospitals; they were thus made responsible for the full spectrum of health services. This reorganization not only provided the opportunity to integrate psychiatric and somatic care, but also stimulated the transfer of psychiatry from mental hospitals into community care facilities. These developments were paralleled by a serious effort to develop facilities for the aged and the chronic sick; in 1968, the goal was to have no less than fifty-five beds per thousand for all people over seventy years of age. However, while the long-term care facilities were a county council responsibility, the homes for the aged were the responsibility of the primary communities. This allocation caused some overlap, which was eventually resolved by a fully comprehensive strategy.

In the Netherlands, catastrophic risks insurance covering the entire population was introduced in 1967 to supplement the existing scheme in the case of prolonged physical or mental illness. By providing reimbursement for extended care of geriatric patients, the mentally retarded, and those with prolonged illnesses, this program created an enormous incentive to improve facilities. The provider community, in particular the nursing homes, responded with a rapid development of well-equipped and well-staffed facilities. Although a number of countries had predicted cost-savings as a result of transferring patients to long-term care institutions, in the Netherlands such savings were not impressive. The Dutch experience with the 1967 Exceptional Medical Expenses Act showed that extended-care facilities, if properly equipped and staffed, have per diem costs nearly as high as acute short-term hospitals of comparable size (Nationaal Ziekenhuis Instituut 1974). During the same period, the Dutch government subsidized many experiments in preventive activities, community mental health centers, and neighborhood health centers, searching for feasible solutions for these neglected areas. Eventually, just as in England and Wales and Sweden, a comprehensive strategy was to emerge.

Because of World War II reconstruction needs, the Federal Republic of Germany was a relative latecomer to the hospital boom of the sixties. Solutions to the problems of the neglected areas of health care had to be delayed, but the problems were nevertheless openly discussed by the media, political groups, and interested parties. While affirmative action was postponed, therefore, until the early seventies (and partly as a result of political developments), when the Germans did begin to deal with these problems, they began immediately to consider a comprehensive approach, rather than employing the stopgap measures tried earlier in other countries.

Developments in France have been less extensive than in the other countries. However, the French have done some experiments with sectorized mental health care, in which defined geographical areas are covered by a structured, comprehensive mental health care service.

Toward a Comprehensive and Integrated System

From the mid-sixties on, the fragmented and often uncoordinated nature of developments in health care became more and more apparent. Strategies focusing on individual components of the health care system—for example, hospitals or mental health or care for chronically ill—gradually gave way to a more comprehensive assessment of the country's total health care needs, leading toward formulation of overall plans for a comprehensive health care system in the decades to come. Coordination of all the components of the health care system, and shifts emphasizing the priority of primary care and the de-institutionalization of care, became very important. Thus, a stopgap strategy gave way to an adaptive strategy, usually in two stages, with the timing in each country depending on its particular range of possibilities.

The emerging comprehensive approach represented a broader application of the principle of equity on which the introduction of health insurance had originally been based. This comprehensiveness was being applied to the supply side of the health care equation, by improving the mix and distribution of resources, rather than to the benefit packages, which already offered all-encompassing entitlement to virtually the entire population of the five countries under study. Thus, the shift to a comprehensive approach also implied much more extensive health care resources development.

The first stage in the introduction of the comprehensive approach was the coordination of independently operating units within a single sector of the health care system. The best examples of this approach are the many attempts—not always successful—to program general hospitals with a view to coordinated action. This programming usually involved either a regionalization scheme, a hierarchization scheme, or both. Sometimes only parts of the hospitals were involved—for example, expensive medical apparatus, emergency care services, or cardiac units—while other times this regionalization and hierarchization also involved other health care institutions, such as mental health and mental care centers, chronic care centers, and health centers.

The second stage in the comprehensive approach was the promotion of a proper balance between the different components of the health care system, usually within the context of a previously developed hospital regionalization scheme. It became important to achieve a high degree of integration among these components because, on the one hand, the cost-effectiveness of individual components, like inpatient facilities, was being questioned, while, on the other hand, gaps and barriers between preventive and curative care, and between somatic and mental care, were becoming increasingly apparent and distressing.

Sweden, England and Wales, and France embraced the notion of a comprehensive hospital program at the beginning of the sixties. In Sweden, the concept of planning hospital organization for a county was born at the beginning of the 1930s. Nevertheless, only when the hospital boom ended in Sweden, revealing a lack of cooperation and misplaced investments, was a Royal Commission on Regionalization of Health Services set up, which in 1960 recommended a completely regionalized, hierarchical hospital system. During the implementation of this system, planning instruments were developed in a cooperative effort between providers—county councils—and central governmental authorities; these instruments permitted the second stage of the comprehensive approach to be achieved in 1973.

In 1973 the Swedish National Board of Health and Welfare issued a comprehensive and integrated health service plan for the 1980s, placing great emphasis on primary care, with 80 percent of ambulatory physician contacts and 65 percent of long-term (nursing home) care, as well as all preventive and dental care, to be offered as much as possible in community-based health centers. In this plan, Sweden departed from its long tradition of hospital-centered care. By creating common boundaries for health areas and administrative areas, the plan seeks to optimize all health care services, in particular primary care services, within each geographic area. Further steps are currently being taken, both politically and technically, to integrate these health care services with the social services available in each region. Though hospitals in England and Wales had virtually the same type of administrative structure as hospitals in Sweden—administration by so-called local authorities—the authorities in Britain were generally too small and too poor, compared with the Swedish county councils, to keep their own hospitals in operation, and were therefore losing ground to the voluntary hospitals. When, as a result of the Second World War, most of Britain's hospitals were nationalized and their administration turned over to regional hospital boards, the hospital system entered a period of "patching and making do." A comprehensive approach was introduced only with the 1962 Hospital Plan. Subsequent evaluation of the National Health Service revealed that the second stage of the comprehensive approach was also badly needed. Indeed, the 1973 reorganization of the National Health Service, which has set an example for this second stage for other European countries, was dominated by the desire to weld the existing tripartite system (hospital services, local authority health services, and general medical services) into an integrated service structured to serve areas whose boundaries were conterminous with those of newly established local authorities. This conterminosity permitted the social services under local authority responsibility to be coordinated with the health services under area health authority responsibility, with both serving the same population group.

In France the drive toward a comprehensive approach, although initiated at roughly the same time as in Sweden and England and Wales, unfortunately suffered a false start. A regionalization and hierarchization scheme were both included in the 1958 Hospital Legislation Reforms, but the necessary change failed to result. Two reasons can be identified: first, the 1958 reforms paid unsufficient attention to the important private sector, which constituted a full 30 percent of French health services; and second, the reform was not accompanied by the legal and administrative instruments necessary to implement it. This second drawback was dealt with in subsequent years, first, by dividing the departments into psychiatric sectors in 1960, second, by formulating directives leading to regionalization in the Fifth Plan, and finally, through the hospital facilities chart of 1968, which combined an inventory of existing hospitals with an estimate of needed facilities, both presented in terms of geographic location.

Not until 1970, however, was major action taken in France. The 1970 reform not only acknowledged the private sector role in a public-private partnership, but also instituted the second stage of the comprehensive approach. The hospital facilities chart was developed to embrace the concept of a health services chart, ultimately encompassing types of health care provision other than just acute care hospital beds.

The first stage of comprehensiveness (single-component coordination) was advocated in the Netherlands in the 1966 Report on National Health Care; but only in 1971 did the Hospital Provision Act create a single national hospital plan. Unfortunately, this plan proved too ambitious, since adequate implementation instruments, such as defined population areas, were lacking. In fact, from the moment the law was enacted, some were suggesting that the original scheme should be replaced by a more realistic plan that would encompass the second stage of the comprehensive approach (multiple components coordination). Thus, the Dutch Policy Proposal on the Structure of the Health Care System, issued in 1974, reflected the same concerns as the 1973 Swedish plan. But since the Dutch government has less control over its health care system, more substantial changes are necessary in the Netherlands than in Sweden to achieve regionalization and hierarchization of health care.

In Germany, the Hospital Finance Act of 1972 was, strictly speaking, concerned only with the first stage leading to a comprehensive approach: the coordinated development of hospital care facilities. However, several articles of the act implied considerably more planning intervention, at the discretion of the individual states. Thus, the question of how to expand into a fully comprehensive approach was in fact touched on. Many position papers have since been published by interested parties, but the actual accomplishments of the different states have been rather limited and divergent. The hierarchization of hospital facilities is not yet widely accepted, and has even been opposed in certain states on the grounds that it would encourage discrimination between "first class" and "second class" hospitals. In Germany, the question of manpower seems to be the stumbling block in moving into the second stage of the comprehensive approach. For example, the bill to alter the relationships between sickness funds and sickness funds affiliated physicians is currently encountering difficulties in the Bundesrat.

Interestingly, in each of the countries the official milestones in the move toward comprehensiveness are clustered around the year 1973. This could lead to the false impression that the countries were aligned and in phase with each other; however, although major events occurred in each country at roughly the same time, the actual pace of subsequent progress has varied considerably. In England and Wales, 1973 saw the first full implementation of a comprehensive integrated health service that had been discussed for nearly a decade. Although the Swedish plan for a comprehensive health care system, issued in 1973, is still being discussed, it does represent a substantial start towards comprehensiveness, since it builds on existing interrelated components. While the 1974 Dutch policy proposal is also an explicit government commitment to the integrated approach, progress towards real legal, administrative, and resource changes is gradual. In Germany and in France, the comprehensive approach is still being discussed largely in the context of hospital-oriented legislative reforms (the 1972 reform in Germany and the 1970 reform in France) with, so far, no formulation of a comprehensive plan.

These differences among the countries can be explained to some extent by two factors. First, in Sweden and England and Wales, the early development of regionalized hospital services providing care for a defined geographical area has been of considerable advantage in the implementation of balanced and integrated comprehensive health services. Meanwhile, in France, the Netherlands, and the Federal Republic of Germany, the main thrust in health service development still springs from the benefits provided by social insurance and the resulting financial support. In these countries, an overall plan can emerge less easily, since the mandate to develop such plans has not been explicitly given to the social insurance agencies, and the national health ministries have traditionally had a relatively weak position within a provider-dominated health care system.

Medical Manpower: The Crucial Resource

In moving very gradually toward integrated comprehensive health care systems (structured into area-related balanced and coordinated provision of primary-care, inpatient care, extended care, preventive services, and social welfare), all the countries began to realize that it was essential to have the right numbers of doctors with the right mix of medical skills at the right points in the system. The medical manpower needed to implement the comprehensive health care plans did not seem to match the existing spatial and functional distribution of established physicians and the numbers and types of new physicians emerging from the educational institutions. The assessments were by and large based on crude approximations, because of a substantial lack of human resources statistics and manpower planning methodology. This manpower planning had failed to develop for three main reasons.

First, although medical manpower had been acclaimed as the key resource in the delivery of health care, the emphasis in planning, organization, and accounting had been on physical resources, a reflection of the earlier preoccupation with hospitals.

Second, there was the question of the medical profession's long-established freedom of action. In aiming to affect the number, distribution, and utilization of physicians, manpower planning was at odds with the professional freedoms that had been established early in the history of the national health programs. Moreover, in each country the physicians constituted one of the few well-organized groups of highly trained individuals who were influential enough to protect the professional freedoms that were, to them, fundamental.

Finally, the instruments needed for manpower planning were lacking. Only when the medical profession acknowledged shortages or surpluses were they willing to agree to an analysis of the manpower situation. Such analysis is a fundamental prerequisite to the development of sensitive planning tools. Each of the countries, in its own way, did make some early moves in the field of medical manpower planning. When the German national health program was reviewed in 1913, a ratio of one physician to every 1,350 subscribers was introduced in the program, and it was determined which doctors would be allowed to treat subscribers of which sickness fund. Reaction against this stipulation was immediate: the doctors went on strike, and the medical profession started to organize. As a result, by 1931 the German medical profession had clearly established itself as a free enterprise profession, subject to only very limited, primarily token, planning stipulations. Thus, though the profession acceded to the professional review regulation included in the 1931 agreement, as stated earlier, this regulation had limited effects, partly because of the rudimentary methodology, but also because of the physicians' strategy of preventing genuine outside involvement, and because the sickness funds were actually more interested in managing their increasing income than in organizing medicine. As late as 1960, the German Supreme Court ruled against physician manpower planning, though the number of medical school students had been limited since the fifties. Only by 1975, when the comprehensive approach was attracting increasing attention, and when increasing discrepancies became apparent in the regional availability of medical services under the free enterprise system did the federal government take the initiative again to propose a law on manpower planning.

In France, following the German example, the medical profession blocked proposals for manpower planning when the 1930 Social Insurance Act was being formulated. The 1958 Reform of Hospital Legislation, though it stressed the hospitals, did touch somewhat on the manpower issue. Planning stipulations were not included, but the free enterprise approach enjoyed by hospital physicians was subjected to certain constraints aimed at improving hospital effectiveness (although exclusively in public hospitals). A hospital career structure was developed, better remuneration conditions were worked out, and full-time medical practice was legally established. In recent years in France, planning efforts have concentrated on medical school enrollments—especially on the size of the second-year medical school class, whereby the first year serves as a screening device—but have left the profession as such untouched. In 1968 the social insurance agencies started to experiment with the establishment of professional activity surveys; and other agencies, especially CREDOC, started to develop a data base of consumer consumption patterns; all of this could help to develop medical manpower planning strategies, but so far, apart from research and information projects, such as the Ministry of Health publication of a "medical establishment chart" in 1976 highlighting the inadequately served regions, no affirmative action has been taken.

The Dutch experience with medical manpower planning deviates from the German and French pattern in one way: from the start, Dutch physicians have been more positively involved in the health insurance business; indeed, many of the voluntary schemes operating before the 1941 Sickness Funds Decree were either run by physicians or had physicians on their boards. As a result of this early involvement, general practitioners were paid on a per capita basis and became the exclusive referral agents to specialists and hospitals. Although serious conflict between the profession and the funds was thus precluded, affirmative action was also delayed, since, apart from the collection of manpower data and manpower research, the initiative remained in the hands of the profession.

However, the 1966 Report on National Health Care, based upon data collected since the Second World War, indicated a shortage of general practitioners and certain specialists in the Netherlands. After 1966, outstanding work was undertaken to research and document the problem—professional activities surveys, general practice morbidity surveys, pilot experiments with group practices, and old-age morbidity surveys—but it was 1971 before decisive action was taken. A 1971 act limiting the number of medical school students (as a result of educational policies unrelated to health policy) was endorsed in the 1974 policy proposal and was followed in 1975 by a plan for general practitioner distribution, to be implemented by the general practitioners on a voluntary basis. If enacted, the 1976 Health Resources Bill will empower the Dutch government to intervene in health manpower supply and its distribution.

Until the 1946 National Health Service Act, the experience of England and Wales ran parallel to the Dutch experience, with the General Medical Council supervising medical education and accreditation. With the 1946 National Health Service Act, however, the government became solely responsible for "the availability of sufficiently and adequately spread medical services." With respect to general practitioners, the authority was delegated to the Medical

Practices Committee, but the government kept its executive power in determining hospital physician posts and career structure. Some blunders occurred because of a lack of manpower planning instruments—especially, of accurate statistics. Notably, in 1957 the Willink Committee reported that the British medical schools would soon be producing too many doctors and that the annual intake of medical students should be reduced by 10 percent. By 1961 the minister of health had to acknowledge a resulting shortage and increase training places by 10 percent (Watkin 1975, p. 227). A solution for these manpower planning difficulties only began to emerge at the beginning of the seventies, by which time the 1973 NHS Reorganization Act allocated the responsibility for medical manpower planning directly to DHSS authorities, where efforts were made to investigate problems and develop planning instruments accordingly (Gunn and Mair 1971).

Sweden stands out among the five countries in having developed a medical manpower strategy that seeks to respond to the needs of the health care system. In fact, Sweden intends to make changes at the foundation of the health care system by changing the content of medical education. The attention given in Sweden to health manpower results from four important factors. In the first place, determining where physicians work and what they do has been a government responsibility since before the turn of the century. As a result, the government early gained experience in matching medical school output to the health services' needs. Second, these early balancing efforts led to prolonged but rigorous debate and study of the controversial issue of physician shortage versus physician surplus, which was alive from 1920 until 1948, when the decision was made to increase the supply of physicians through government action: by raising student intake in existing medical schools, creating new medical schools, and importing foreign-trained doctors. Third, manpower development policies in general, and the objective of matching the output of educational institutions to the manpower needs of the economy, were constant elements of Swedish economic policy from 1932 to 1976, while the Social Democratic government was in power.

Finally, the serious commitment in Sweden to equality in general, as well as the particular commitment of the Social Democrats to this objective, also focused attention on physicians' incomes and sought to equalize them. There was the question of bringing physician incomes in line with other professional incomes, and, within the medical profession, there was the question of a wide range of incomes among specialists, and between junior and senior staff. The 1970 Seven Kronor Reform altered this situation. Replacing potentially high reimbursable fees for outpatient visits with a small standard fee regardless of the services rendered, and putting physicians on salary instead of permitting them to collect fees for outpatient visits, this reform was inspired by the desire for equity of access. It was hoped to encourage patients with modest incomes to seek outpatient care by eliminating the prospect of their having to advance a large sum of money that only later would be reimbursed.

The Seven Kronor Reform was politically feasible because it fulfilled platform promises for equality. In one stroke, economic equality was introduced in three ways: physicians' incomes were brought in line with each other, they were brought in line with the incomes of other professionals, and the last remnants of economic discrimination among patients were virtually abolished (if one can ignore the small percentage of physicians still in private practice in Sweden). Putting physicians on salary resulted in more explicit rules regarding hours of service, overtime and compensation; these in turn led to more detailed manpower utilization statistics.

The planning of medical manpower in Sweden is no longer a matter merely of projecting required numbers of doctors. The detailed medical manpower requirements formulated at the county council level, following guidelines derived from the national health policy, are translated at the national level into demands to be met both quantitatively and qualitatively by the educational system. The formulation of these demands takes place in formal consultation between the National Board of Health and Welfare and the Office of the Chancellor of the Swedish Universities. None of the other countries has progressed so far as Sweden in health manpower planning. All the countries have made modest attempts to reorient the training of general practitioners, preparing them for a key role in primary care, but so far, only Sweden has introduced specialist training in primary care. When the need for more emphasis on behavioral sciences in the medical curriculum and the importance of primary care were eventually acknowledged everywhere in the late 1960s, it was also recognized that these shifts would have to be initiated virtually in a vacuum, in opposition to an enormous hospital-centered power base.

The strong emphasis on primary care in comprehensive health care plans and policy proposals is at odds with the limited effort made by the academic establishment to prepare physicians for new roles in health care delivery. For instance, the current training efforts to produce primary care physicians in the Dutch or Swedish universities (where a strong hospital and research bias still prevails) may very well fall short of the needs expressed in ambitious government policy proposals.

Beyond the Traditional Resources

The shift over the years from the original policy of ensuring access to physicians' services to the current policy of comprehensive national health care planning not only involves further development of certain existing resources, but has also highlighted the need for new types of resources. Health facilities, health technology, biomedical knowledge, and health manpower are all necessary; but in designing and implementing a comprehensive health care system—however differently this may be defined from one country to another—resources such as information, vital statistics, health resources data, and health services research become vital. They in turn entail managerial and systems resources, involving many interdependent units and health care settings.

The emergence of health care managers, that is, professionals in such disciplines as health statistics, health care planning, and hospital administration, has received less attention in Europe than in the United States. In Europe, graduate training in health statistics and epidemiology is at present available only at the London School of Hygiene and at the French National School of Public Health in Rennes. No regular training program in health planning is offered in any of the countries under study, although the World Health Organization has sponsored ad hoc courses that were jointly organized by Sweden and the USSR. Training for hospital administration was nonexistent in Europe until 1956, when the University of Manchester introduced the first European hospital management program. A survey made by Jan Blanpain in 1970 at the request of the World Health Organization showed that there were then only twelve graduate and undergraduate programs in the countries under study, of which eight were in the United Kingdom and one in each of the other countries (World Health Organization 1972). In the United

States, whose population in 1973 was only slightly higher than the aggregated populations of the five countries, there were seventy-seven graduate and thirty-one undergraduate programs in health administration and planning (Austin, Ball, and Clark 1975).

The low esteem in which management is held in Europe is probably one of the reasons for this difference. In Europe management as a profession is less appreciated than in the United States, and the possibility of training managers through formal educational processes is accepted only reluctantly. The American attitude toward management is probably related to the greater value that American society accords to entrepreneurial, free-market ideology. In Europe management tends to be viewed as a limited role, consisting of housekeeping, administering accounts, making budgets, and preparing personnel rosters; all this carries nasty connotations of the trivial, the bureaucratic, and the like. However, in 1967 Jean-Jacques Servan-Schreiber shocked a great many Europeans by declaring in his best-seller *Le défi Americain* ("The American Challenge") that the so-called technological gap between the U.S. and Europe, and the takeover by American multinationals of Europe's industries, was not so much a question of superior and innovative technology, but more a matter of managerial superiority (Servan-Schreiber 1967). In contrast, it is fair to remark that the strong American emphasis on the accountability of the health manager, and on his role as an advocate of the interests of the community, has to some degree been pre-empted in Europe by more progressive social policies and by the dominance of the medical profession. In the United States, managers at the lower echelons of the health care system are responsible for developments that in European countries result from overall government policies, or from the simple fact of a more homogenous population that values health very highly and is willing to support all social endeavors and health policies adopted by government. It is an open question whether it is socially efficient and desirable for lower-echelon health care administrators in the United States to be expected to forge new structures and to overhaul the organization so that it genuinely meets the needs of the population.

In Europe the medical profession constantly interferes with operational management, through clinical autonomy in diagnostic and therapeutic interventions; the exclusion of laymen from medical disciplinary matters; strong representation of professional interests in statutory and advisory agencies, with, in many cases, overriding veto power; and collective bargaining through intricate negotiating structures, usually carried on with authorities at levels above the employing authorities. All these factors limit and erode the role of management at the operational level, and possess the constant danger of reducing it to sheer housekeeping. Ironically, the dominance of the medical profession makes the managerial role at the corporate level even more complex. The planning and developmental strategies must be acceptable to and compatible with the physician's special position as one of the system's main production factors.

At present, France offers, through its National School of Public Health, a training program for civil servants preparing for hospital management careers. The absence of public health schools in the Federal Republic of Germany, the Netherlands, and to some extent in Sweden (where a Nordic School of Public Health, with very limited teaching activities, serves the whole of Scandinavia) partly explains the limited efforts in health management education in these countries. Business management schools have also developed only modestly in these countries. Thus, the settings in which health services administration training has traditionally developed in the United States are virtually nonexistent.

By and large, England and Wales have opted for ongoing training of health managers, by providing progressive stages of responsibility in conjunction with supervised practical experience alternating with periods of academic instruction. A potentially important new managerial resource has begun to be recognized in England and Wales: specialists in community medicine. As specialized medical administrators, they are expected to play a key role in health care planning, in particular by assessing health care needs and translating them into coordinated efforts for health care provision (Gatherer 1971, p. 95). Special training in community medicine is already available at the British schools of public health. Among its various objectives, the 1973 NHS reorganization placed great emphasis on improving management. Special attention was paid to management arrangements, organizational structures, lines of communication, delegation of authority, and consensus management.

Coping with the sheer size and complexities of the emerging comprehensive health care systems requires that the focus of health management education shift to the senior managers. While the few European programs in health management are still mainly geared towards producing managers at the operational level, such as hospital administrators, future priorities must turn towards the development, through education and continuing education, of managers at higher levels. A major challenge confronting those educating and training senior health managers is to refute the widespread conviction that sound judgment can be developed only through experience. The education of health managers must embody an epidemiological perspective on health and disease, whereby the focus is shifted from institutions to populations, and whereby outcomes and social impact are more important than producing outputs. Senior managers must be trained to apply epidemiological concepts and techniques. At the same time the future senior manager should be introduced to cure and care processes as the patient encounters them. Only through an understanding of clinical decision-making and of the dynamics of the sociocultural context in which patients interact with the providers of care will managers be able to effect change so as to meet population needs in an epidemiological perspective.

These considerations have only recently come under discussion in the survey countries and only within limited circles. The universities and medical teaching centers have so far failed to provide leadership and have not allocated the needed resources to develop advanced management education for the health sector. In the United States, philanthropic foundations like the Kellogg Foundation and the Milbank Foundation have been extremely important in introducing and developing university-based graduate and postgraduate education in health management and health planning. Among the European countries studied, however, only England and Wales have similar philanthropic support. In an attempt to realize their important commitment to raise the managerial capacity of the National Health Service, the Nuffield Provincial Hospitals Trust and the King's Fund joined forces in 1975 in the Working Party on the Education and Training of Senior Managers, which in January 1977 submitted its final draft report. This report stressed an innovative rather than a reactive strategy, whereby the varying needs of the professions involved in health management would be met specifically through the development of corporate management perspective and competence. It also proposed a closer interaction between the universities and the National Health Service, in which the universities would provide management education to meet the managerial needs of the health care system, while the health care system would recognize the universities' need for a health services research base in the community and the NHS (Working Party 1977). In light of the emerging importance of health care managers, the government use of management consulting firms in the design of comprehensive health care policies is an interesting development. Management consulting firms have been less involved in the problems of hospital operations and capital investment management in Europe than in the United States. Nevertheless, McKinsey and Company was hired during the preliminary work for the 1973 Reorganization of the National Health Service in the United Kingdom and has been active in other European countries as well (Maxwell 1976, p. 5). Comparable commercial firms were called upon in the Netherlands during the preparation of the 1974 Policy Proposal on the Structure of Health Care.

The need for health care information and for planning methods, management systems, resource allocation techniques, and operations research has led to the creation of special purpose organizations oriented toward management, information or health services research. In each of the five countries, the appropriate ministry, of health or of social affairs, has strengthened its existing information-oriented branch or division or created special divisions under its direct control, such as the Institute for Social Medicine and Epidemiology of the Federal Health Bureau, established in 1969 in Germany, or the Planning, Programming, and Budgeting System and Operations Research Section, created in 1970 in the French Ministry of Health.

These new types of resources have also been developed outside government institutions. A national institute or center devoted to hospital management and research was established using voluntary contributions from hospital associations in the Federal Republic of Germany in Dusseldorf in 1953 and in the Netherlands at Utrecht in 1968. In England and Wales the King's Fund operates a hospital center comparable to the Dutch and German Institutes. In France, CREDOC, which was established in 1954 as a semivoluntary organization, plays a national role in studies on health economics and health care utilization.

In all the countries, universities, primarily through traditional research support, have initiated health services research. Focused on organizational, financial, and other aspects of health care delivery, this research has been modest in volume when compared to biomedical research. In a survey of Belgium, France, the Federal Republic of Germany, and the Netherlands, made at the request of the Nuffield Provincial Hospitals Trust, Blanpain and Delesie found in 1976 that health services research expenditures (inside and outside universities) as a percentage of total health research expenditures, were 6.5 percent in the Netherlands, 2.4 percent in France, and 1.4 percent in the Federal Republic of Germany (Blanpain and Delesie 1976). In the United Kingdom, the Nuffield Provincial Hospitals Trust has played a special role in sponsoring and guiding university health services research, with the result that a stream of outstanding publications has appeared. The trust's pioneering efforts were eventually supplemented by substantial financial resources from the Department of Health and Social Security, which allocated some two million pounds to health services research in 1970 (Cohen 1971, p. 3).

Thus, the role of health services research in solving operational and resource allocation problems and in contributing to health policy formulation is discussed much more in England and Wales than in the other countries studied. The evaluation of previous research and the formulation of a health services research strategy, which took place at a 1974 Oxford meeting sponsored by the Nuffield Trust, have no parallel so far in the other countries (McLachlan 1974). In Sweden, however, SPRI, created jointly by the Federation of County Councils and the National Board of Health and Social Welfare in 1968, has developed an important planning, research, and development capacity, highly oriented towards demonstration and implementation. Only two of the countries, England and Wales and the Netherlands, have so far formulated a specific term expressing concisely the concept of research devoted to organizational or other aspects of health care. The terms "health services research," in England and Wales, and *Gezondheidsonderzoek,* in the Netherlands, represent a "named-idea," which, according to De Bono, is an advanced stage in the efficiency of thinking and communication. The other countries, where a sentence is needed to express the concept, are still at the stage of what De Bono calls a "bundle-idea" (De Bono 1976, p. 46). This difference is one of the main indications that health services research is less visible in those three countries. In each country, a mutually productive relationship can now be observed between hospital or health care managers in the field, on the one hand, and hospital or health care information, management, and research organizations, on the other. Each serves the other as a training ground. The information capability and research results, however, vary. Sweden is the forerunner with respect to information, but, except for planning methodology, health services research results are rather limited. England is the forerunner in health services research results, but somewhat lacking in information capability. In the Netherlands, information and research capability are equally balanced. French information and research capability is heavily oriented towards macro-economics, while the Federal Republic of Germany is lagging in both information and research capability (Blanpain and Delesie 1976).

The Imperatives of Restraint

Over the years since health insurance was introduced, there has been a general increase in both the quantity and the quality of health resources, whether this increase was pursued directly or resulted indirectly from having more money available for health care. Now this trend toward improving health "at any cost" is being questioned and may be halted or even reversed as future plans develop.

Cost-containment is undoubtedly the dominant force behind this change. All five countries, except, to a certain extent, England and Wales, have witnessed a substantial rise in the percentage of GNP spent on health and in per capita expenditure for health. In the Netherlands between 1968 and 1972 the percentage of GNP devoted to health services rose from 5.9 percent to 7.3 percent, and in Sweden between 1969 and 1970 it rose from 6.4 percent to 7 percent (Maxwell 1976, p. 7). In those countries that rely on social insurance to finance health care, employer and employee contributions are reaching the limits of public acceptability, and are provoking discontent among employers in labor-intensive industries, who have to contribute much more than employers in capital-intensive industries.

The prolonged economic recession of the seventies, with slower growth of GNP, has further strengthened the conviction that health care costs must be contained. However, cost-containment for health care probably would not in itself change health care strategies significantly were other important issues not also involved.

One issue that has stimulated further investigation is the question of efficiency. The development of new and different health resources, such as management, information, and research resources, has not only led to new developments in health care delivery, but has also highlighted the drawbacks of the traditional approaches. The hospital-oriented research institutes are a significant example. Although they were established specifically to increase hospital efficiency, their work did more to reveal shortcomings in the hospital-based system than to resolve problems of inefficiency.

Statistics on the health care delivery system reveal wide discrepancies in resource utilization and consumption among care settings, provider groups, consumer groups, and national regions. By the end of the sixties, these discrepancies were clearly outlined. In reaction, there was a surge of research—sometimes of questionable value—aimed at tracing out the acceptable or average patterns of resource utilization and resource consumption: beds per thousand; average lengths of stay; optimal hospital size; nursing personnel per hundred beds; acceptable depreciation costs; and so forth. But much of this work was to little avail. Either the norms were too insensitive, too rigid, or too limited to guarantee successful implementation, or the development of the health care setting to which they applied had gained so much momentum that no norm-setting could stop it in its tracks. Other, more comprehensive approaches became mandatory, and new questions emerged. For example, there is the rapidly spreading belief (supported by some evidence, like reduced age-specific life expectancies) that the enormous increase in health care expenditure has not been responsible for significant improvements in health status. Through an analysis of mortality figures dating back to the eighteenth century McKeown, among others, has weakened the conviction that the improvement of health and life-expectancy over the centuries has been due primarily to medical intervention: "This concept is not in accord with past experience. The improvement of health during the past three centuries was due essentially to provision of food, protection from hazards and limitation of numbers; medical science and services made an important contribution to the control of hazards but only a limited one through immunization and therapy" (McKeown 1976, p. 178).

Thus, the continuing tendency to improve the qualifications of health care workers and to raise the levels of capital investment, with the result that doctors and facilities have become overqualified or overequipped to deal with common medical problems, compounded by the trend for human problems previously dealt with outside the realm of medicine to be brought increasingly into the health domain, is being discussed and investigated. The cost-effectiveness of certain expensive medical interventions is being questioned, and a mandatory, systematic appraisal of the effectiveness of diagnostic and therapeutic procedures is repeatedly proposed. The varying effectiveness of a wide range of approaches to given health care problems is similarly being scrutinized. Cochrane's 1972 publication *Effectiveness and Efficiency,* in which he suggests a more systematic use of randomized clinical trials of medical treatments, has been translated in several languages and is cited and quoted again and again (Cochrane 1972). In the same vein, the 1975 Excerpta Medica Award was given in Amsterdam to a Danish researcher, Dr. Juhl, who was singled out among many candidates for his work on randomized clinical trails in gastroenterology (Davis 1976). From time to time, the health care establishment is accused of indulging in unnecessary costly and dangerous practices, as in Ivan Illich's bestseller *Medical Nemesis* (Illich 1975).

Closely related to these doubts about the traditionally unquestioned claim for more health care resources is the growing conviction that approaches other than health services may be able to deal effectively with certain health problems. Traffic safety programs, including speed limits, enforced use of safety belts, and stringent anti-alcohol measures, have already proved more cost effective in reducing automobile fatalities than accident treatment and rehabilitation programs have been.

Thus, the problems of rising costs and limited effectiveness have been approached in different ways. One approach is utilization control. In England and Wales and the Netherlands, national "hospital discharge abstracts analysis systems" have been developed, providing, in principle, a self-regulatory monitoring device for hospital utilization control. However, the absence of a traditional medical staff organization to implement the method, and the prevailing climate of noninterference in clinical judgment, hindered the effective use of such monitoring. At the end of 1976 the Dutch Specialists Association and the Medical Association for the Promotion of Hospital Care issued an important joint statement committing these two important groups and their membership to a voluntary nationwide medical audit and utilization control program in general hospitals (Landelijke Specialisten Vereniging 1976). In a recent publication, Gordon McLachlan reveals the fascinating range of initiatives that have been taken in the United Kingdom in the domain of medical audit and quality assurance, but he expresses a pointed hope for the growth of a more "sympathetic atmosphere" within the profession with respect to the monitoring of health care quality (McLachlan 1976).

In France, utilization statistics on individual providers and consumers, an updated version of the 1931 German approach, have recently been introduced. Although agreed upon in principle, this approach has so far been implemented only on an experimental basis, mainly because the profession remains sensitive to such efforts. Sweden, which among the five countries definitely has the most systematic and up-to-date view of how, by whom, and for what its health services are utilized, is gradually shifting away from post-factum utilization control, which by its very nature offers limited options for improving the situation—one can either create financial disincentives against misutilization (the German approach), or try to educate people toward more proper utilization (the Dutch approach). The Swedish approach now appears to be to tackle cost-containment within a larger framework. From draft documents discussed at SPRI, the National Board of Health and Welfare and SPRI appear to be promoting so-called medical care programs. These consist of directives and guidelines about providing patient care for given diseases in given care settings. What some may object to as cookbook medicine is being carefully explored, discussed, and formulated into prescribed lines of action. Consensus among professionals is sought, as is coordination with training programs, so that a high degree of consistency can be achieved. The medical programs are primarily geared toward medical conditions that are highly prevalent, consume substantial resources, and can be identified with relative certainty.

By introducing medical programs, the Swedes expect to shift the burden of proof for ineffective and inefficient use of resources from retrospective audit to the prospective responsibility of the medical profession as a whole, and thus to eliminate, in advance and in agreement, questionable practices and wastes of resources. This development, which attempts to switch from corrective feedback through peer review to direct guidance through peer consensus, is an enormously important social experiment and is worth following closely. Of course, such a development is possible in Sweden because of the high degree of mutual respect and understanding that exists between the medical profession and government there.

A second major avenue for coping with rising costs and ensuring cost-effectiveness is control on the supply side of health services.

This is being pursued in many directions: de-institutionalization of health care, primarily by reorienting and strengthening the primary care level, is high on the agenda in all the countries, but especially England and Wales, the Netherlands, and Sweden. Apart from providing care in more appropriate settings (in terms of continuity in providers, human dignity, and minimum disruption of social contacts), one of the major assumptions underlying the new interest in primary care is the potential for cost-containment in avoiding expensive inpatient care. However, there is so far little or no documented evidence to show that better primary care will result in reduced costs.

A corollary to this is the reduction of inpatient care facilities, primarily in acute short-term hospitals. England and Wales and the Netherlands are highly committed to such reductions, at present more than the other countries. A shift towards ambulatory care and more extended-care facilities underlies this policy. As already mentioned, the policy depends on the assumption that ambulatory care will prove less costly. As to the cost-containing effect of providing extended care in special extended-care facilities rather than short-term hospitals, the Dutch experience with the 1967 Exceptional Medical Expenses Act invites caution.

Control of the supply of doctors has been introduced in all the countries under study. Control on expensive health care technology is another emerging approach towards cost-containment. In England and Wales and Sweden, this control is an aspect of budgeting controls on capital investment; the governments in the countries also determine those settings in the health care system where expensive technology will be concentrated. In France, the Netherlands, and the Federal Republic of Germany, investment in expensive health technology is becoming subject to planning, certification-of-need, and licensing. The Dutch state secretary for health is hoping that, by combining controls on the supply of health care resources with strict controls on all fees and prices in the provision of health care, the cost-explosion will be brought under control. This belief underlies his introduction of a Health Resources Bill and a Health Tariffs Bill at the end of 1976. However, Dutch organized medicine is concerned about these restraint policies and may oppose them. On December 10, 1976, the Dutch Specialists Association devoted its entire annual assembly in Utrecht to the cost-containment issue. The specialists expressed extreme concern over the government plans, and they issued a statement that they would consider the government bills only as temporary measures inspired by the prevailing economic crisis. The specialists said that a reduction in hospital capacity would be equivalent to the senseless destruction of the weaving machines in Great Britain at the start of the industrial revolution.

German free-practicing physicians started go-slow actions in February 1977 to protest government plans to contain health care costs. These plans included a proposal to limit increases in physician income to the rate of growth of the GNP and to make the medical profession responsible for drug costs that increased beyond a certain percentage. Such measures are viewed by the medical profession as virtually state medicine (*Der Spiegel* 1977).

A final avenue for cost-containment is through changes in consumer demand for health services. A new and more important role is visualized for health education in a two-pronged approach that is intended to increase an individual's sense of responsibility about his own health and induce him to use health services more judiciously. The health care consumer might receive more attention and become an important health care resource if the growing conviction that health is largely a behavioral and environmental problem actually were to be acted upon. So far, recognition of the need to increase an individual's responsibility for his own health and to influence environmental factors and hazards, rather than simply investing in costly health services, has remained largely academic. The comprehensive health care plans that England and Wales, Sweden and the Netherlands have already formulated still focus on the strengthening of health services and on the delivery of personal health care, although they express an interest in coordinated health and social services. The challenge for the future will be to enlarge these plans to include lifestyle programs, on the one hand, and environmental programs on the other, with a more balanced and eventually reduced investment in health services development.

8 | The Role of Government

Government actions have obviously been an important influence in the evolution of national health programs. The concluding section of our analysis highlights major areas in which government has intervened—especially, the financing of health care—and the different modes of government action taken, emphasizing the distinction between actions at the national or sub-national level.

The Financing of Health Care

Although in all five countries the financing of national health programs was introduced to make access to health care independent of a patient's financial means, in each case this was accomplished at the start through regulations designed to minimize socially and politically unacceptable inequities rather than through sweeping reforms aimed at optimizing actual health care delivery. The impulse to make health care accessible to everyone stemmed from the principle of equity that had been at work in all five countries since the very beginning of national health insurance. During the development of their national health insurance programs, some countries experienced a continuous process of increasing democratization that reinforced this principle of equity. Even though four of the five countries endured the World War II experiences that resulted, in Eastern Europe, in a totalitarian approach under the motto of collective ownership of the means of production, in the Western European countries a fundamentally democratic orientation still exists. Those mandatory programs that have emerged—the National Health Service in England and Wales, the health care facilities chart in France, the county hospitals in Sweden—are all based on the cooperation of consumers and providers. However, this democratization has not, in general, led to a radical overhaul of the health care delivery system itself, for several reasons.

The first reason is primarily historic. Upon the introduction of its national health program, each country was confronted with a network of existing insurance schemes, in many cases linked to political power blocks. These blocks could not be ignored; they had to be integrated through financial incentives and regulatory measures. A second reason was the growing power of the medical profession, because of the increasing status of medical science and the strengthened position of organized medicine. The national health program and its financial incentives had to respect the province of medical practice and to limit constraints on free development of this practice.

Thus, when national health insurance was introduced, government involvement was tolerated only in administration and regulation, not in management or direction. Until recently, most national health program data, including financial data, were geared towards administering and controlling individual parts of the health service, rather than managing and running the entire national health program.

Because government involvement had to be conciliatory, partial, and regulatory, the financing of the national health program in the countries studied was characterized by several distinctive features. First, it embodied—to varying degrees—a principle of complementarity, in which the national government was to provide money only when private and local money proved deficient. This public money varied from token subsidies for the development of particular health care experiments, as in the Netherlands, to the 40-percent financing of public hospitals in France, to the almost totally subsidized national health service in England and Wales. The extent to which funds from the national government support the components of the national health program is a function of each country's historical development and political priorities; no general rule is applicable. In all cases, however, public finances catalyze resource development: they accelerate or decelerate trends whose original momentum comes from social developments, political decisions, or the particular requests of lobbying groups.

A second common feature of each country's national health finance policy was the initial concentration on health care benefits and their accessibility, before dealing with health care provision and availability. Sweden was an exception to this rule, since geographical constraints—a very low population density—forced it to consider provision before benefits. All the other countries went through a period in which increasing financial means were used primarily to expand national health program coverage by enlarging the population group entitled, by extending benefits, or by facilitating procedures such as third party payment. One characteristic of this process was that for a long time the cabinet member most important to the national health program was not the minister of public health but the minister responsible for social affairs or social security. Unfortunately, when executive and administrative responsibilities are divided between two ministers, the accurate matching of health resources to the provision of benefits becomes very difficult. The Netherlands, France, and the Federal Republic of Germany have all experienced these problems, and are only just beginning to establish constructive relationships between the two areas of responsibility.

This emphasis on benefits gave significant leverage to the national health insurance funds in the Federal Republic of Germany, France, and the Netherlands. Their control of a rapidly increasing cash flow gave them considerable influence in the day-to-day running of the national health program. Only when this trend began to level off did health care provision and availability begin to receive attention. The pattern of manipulating national health program financing to compensate for discrepancies in either the access to health care or the availability of health care providers was established early and persisted for a long time. From the start, for instance, the public funds were directed towards diminishing the discrepancies in accessibility to health care which existed between the wage earners and the professions. When financing shifted focus from benefits to availability of health care, the tendency to concentrate on particular discrepancies resulted in certain types of resources being developed out of proportion to the rest of the system. The best example of this is the postwar development of hospitals. Since the development of acute-care hospitals had been halted during the war, and since the medical model in vogue subsequently emphasized their pivotal role, they were in a favored position to argue for funds.

When the regulatory power that went along with the distribution of funds aimed at alleviating discrepancies proved insufficient to ensure a satisfactory distribution, four of the five countries envisioned a mandatory power: Sweden, France, England and Wales, and to some extent the Netherlands. When this mandatory power still proved insufficient (which it usually did because it still applied only to discrepancies within one single benefit or provision component), the countries began to regard finances as the common denominator with which to treat problems in a more comprehensive way. This has resulted finally in the emergence of a new objective: managing the national health program to produce optimal delivery of care, rather than regulating it to minimize discrepancies in the delivery of care. Three countries—England and Wales since the National Health Service Reorganization Act of 1973 and the introduction of the Annual Budget Cycle, Sweden since the establishment of the National Health Planning Council in 1964 and the Permanent Committee on Health Planning in 1971, and the Netherlands since the publication of the 1974 Policy Proposal—seem to be on their way to regarding health finances as a tool for managing the national health program.

Modes of Government Action

Health resources development to a great extent results from the actions taken by agencies, organizations, or institutions dedicated to the creation of given types of resources. Medical schools produce doctors; research institutions produce medical expertise; a resources development fund, like the Special Development Fund operating in France within the Social Security Administration, produces health facilities. Thus government action in resource development also operates mainly through institutionalized developers. As indicated in the discussion of the government role in the provision of health services, two major modes of government action can be distinguished: the regulatory approach and the direct provision approach. All five countries began to regulate private institutionalized developers very early, by granting or by withholding access to general revenue or to health insurance financing. The main developers of health manpower resources are educational institutions: medical schools, schools for nursing and allied personnel, and schools for health care managers. Very early, in 1814 in France and in 1858 in England, national governments began to influence the educational programs by trying to impose standard curricula. This was accomplished even before medical schools were taken over by the central government. Subsequently, the government regulated medical schools and other health educational institutions in recurrent reforms of their curricula. Another aspect of the regulation of health manpower is control of the numbers and the distribution of health care workers. Government can affect this directly in different ways. It can exercise its influence at the very beginning by determining medical school enrollment, or it can act at the end of the educational process through accreditation regulations. In France, the Netherlands, and the Federal Republic of Germany, the government determines the annual intake of students in medical school, and the latter two countries have taken the first legal steps to regulate the distribution of physicians, either geographically or functionally. In England and Wales, the start of the National Health Service was accompanied by measures to redistribute general practitioners more equitably throughout the country by determining over-doctored areas.

As to physical resources, the main developers affected by the government are private profit and nonprofit groups and health insurance agencies. In Sweden and England and Wales, there are very few of these and they are not really affected by government action. The most common mechanism of government action in the other three countries involves a juridical framework within which the nongovernmental hospital developers have to act (in the Federal Republic of Germany, the 1972 Hospital Finance Act; in France, the 1970 Hospital Reform Act; in the Netherlands, the 1971 Hospital Provision Act). The most rigid system exists in France, where no hospital can be built without ministerial approval; in the Federal Republic of Germany, if private groups by-pass hospital plans prepared by the states, they are not eligible for government financial aid. In all three countries, government action is based on a national hospital plan (gradually being replaced by a health facilities plan), with a planning committee advising the government: in the Federal Republic of Germany, the Committee on Questions Concerning the Economic Security of the Hospitals; in France, the National and Regional Hospital Committees; and in the Netherlands, the Council for Hospital Provisions.

A very recent development in the regulatory approach is that it is increasingly intended to diminish hospital development and to encourage the development—mainly through financial support—of primary care programs. This tendency is very clear in the Netherlands, and has begun to emerge, although less prominently, in the Federal Republic of Germany and in France. In France and in the

Netherlands, government intervention explicitly extends to the regulation of expensive health technology, while in the Federal Republic of Germany a great variety of constraints are imposed. With regard to health services research and statistical resources, the governments are tentatively beginning to use regulatory mechanisms to redirect voluntary efforts into more mission-oriented and applications-oriented endeavors.

The second major mode of government action is direct provision of health resources. In each of the five countries, the government has established its own medical schools and other health-related educational institutions. In some cases, medical schools have been established explicitly to affect the supply of physicians (the medical school of Rotterdam in the Netherlands, 1967); in other cases, the objective was to provide equal access to university-based education (the medical school of Maastricht in the Netherlands, 1973).

The firmest government control over medical manpower exists in Sweden. As early as 1920, physician supply was the subject of Swedish government concern. At present, admission to medical schools is regulated by the Central Office of the Chancellor of the Universities. Originally, the chancellor was a university representative; now he is a civil servant. This change represents a subtle shift towards greater government influence over the supply of physicians. Further, in Sweden the government has the prerogative to determine the number and type of physician positions in hospitals and the medical officer corps. Educational planning and the determination of health manpower needs are considered and coordinated in joint consultation between the National Board of Health and Welfare and the Office of the Chancellor of the Universities.

As to the development of physical resources, in England and Sweden the governments have taken over entirely the responsibility for the development of hospitals and health centers. In France and, to a lesser degree, in the Federal Republic of Germany, local authorities have developed hospital resources. The governments of the five countries under study have been especially active in creating medical research or health services research institutions, to the extent even that in some countries, because of existing voluntary institutions, a rather chaotic pattern has emerged. Some of these institutions only study health care, while others have broader research goals.

As for work in health resource development in general, agencies comparable to the Health Resources Fund, established in Canada in

1966 before the implementation of the Canadian Medical Care Insurance Program, or the Health Resources Development Fund, proposed in the Corman-Kennedy bill in the United States (to receive ultimately 5 percent of total income of the health insurance program to be used for improving and increasing health resources), have rarely been established in the countries under study, although a Special Development Fund was created after World War II in France within the Social Security Administration. Rather than using resource development funds, national health programs in Europe have relied on the existing supply of resources to meet changed needs. Health resources development programs have not been instituted, first, because of the underdevelopment of data systems capable of providing information about the variety in existing resources and, second, because, for a long period, there was only a limited social surplus left over after basic needs had been met, so that only the most marginal health resources development was feasible.

Government action in resources development has fallen into roughly three stages of increased intervention: regulation of voluntary developers, regulation of resource supply and distribution, and, finally, direct provision of resources. In relation to most health resources, Sweden and England and Wales have progressed to stage three, while the other three countries are at present moving into stage two.

A further distinction can be drawn between the different levels of government. The countries differ in the roles reserved for the national, subnational, and local government. Generally, decision-making authority is exercised within the framework set at the national level, with one exception: in the Federal Republic of Germany the eleven states (*Länder*) have real legislative power in health care matters, and can legislate insofar as the constitution does not confer specific legislative powers to the federation, or to the extent that the federation does not use its power. But even there power is shifted subtly from the states towards the federation, mainly because of the federation's financial leverage. Nevertheless, the states remain powerful, because one of the two chambers of the Federal Parliament is composed entirely of state representatives.

In all the countries, the national executive offices in matters of health care are the ministries of health. Germany still has separate ministries for health care and health insurance, but the other four countries have merged health care and health insurance under one ministry, although there are sometimes separate administrative boards, as in Sweden. Interestingly, ministries other than the ministry of health are involved in a piecemeal way in the administration of health care in all five countries, mostly for historical reasons.

A distinction exists at the subnational level between functional authorities and geographic authorities. Functional authorities are special mission-oriented bodies that administer and supervise health care services in local or regional health areas. These bodies are appointed, not elected. Geographic authorities have an overall responsibility, including health care matters, for a regional or local area. In general, geographic authorities are democratically elected by the population they serve. The Regional and Area health authorities in England and Wales are examples of functional authorities. In the Federal Republic of Germany, France, and the Netherlands, the geographic authorities, regional or provincial, and the municipal authorities exercise executive health care duties within a broad mandate. The Swedish county councils constitute a mixture of geographic and functional authorities: they are democratically elected, but their mandate is almost exclusively in the health care field. Arguments in favor of functional authorities are that, in principle, they have independent financial resources, so that health resources development does not have to compete with other services. The five countries can be ranked according to the prominence of their subnational level in health resources development, as follows: the Federal Republic of Germany, Sweden, England and Wales, France, and the Netherlands.

The Federal Republic of Germany comes first because it is a federation in which the eleven states were given important health care responsibilities by the constitutional legislation of 1948. These states received responsibility for education and training in universities. Appointments to universities were to be made by the state ministers of education. During the sixties the states founded new medical schools. Different states, in a cooperative effort with health insurance funds, tried to redress the uneven distribution of general practitioners in their area. However, following an amendment to the constitution on May 12, 1969, the federation received the authority to plan national education in a cooperative effort with the states. By 1970, the medical curriculum was reformed at the federal level. In 1975, the federal government again took the initiative, with a proposal aimed at a fair distribution of sickness funds affiliated physicians and a strengthening of suburban and rural medical practice. As to nursing and allied health personnel, the states themselves introduced regulations on their development immediately after World War II. But, from 1957 onwards, the federal government has introduced further regulations (nursing, 1957; medical-technical assistants, 1958; sickness gymnasts, masseurs, 1958).

The states received responsibility for hospital development in 1948, with each state responding very differently. In 1954, the federation intervened for the first time. The minister of economic affairs, using his authority in matters of price control, promulgated instructions to stabilize the hospital bed reimbursement rates. Eventually, this federal price regulation made the hospital financing system totally unworkable. The federation's lack of legal power to solve these financing problems was at the root of the 1969 constitutional amendment. The amendment made possible the Hospital Finance Act of 1972, through which the federal government has finally become involved in physical resources development, in partnership with the states.

The 1948 Königstein Agreement delegated to the states greater responsibility for health research and information resources. In recent years, however, the federal government's coordinating role has increased, partly because the states have been unable to develop a coordinated research policy.

In summary, an equilibrium between states and the federation appears likely in the near future, with the states meeting the demand for medical care in an optimal, efficient, and economic way, and the federal government having responsibility for planning the entire health service.

In Sweden, the subnational level is also very important. Already in 1862 the provision of medical services was gradually being brought under the authority of the county councils, while the central authority remained responsible for planning and supervision. Over the years, the county councils have become responsible for the full spectrum of health services. This extensive county involvement in the provision of health care is also reflected in the financial burden they carry: by 1970, 67 percent of Sweden's total health care costs were covered through the county councils' special taxation. Since 1920, the counties have been grouped into the powerful Federation of County Councils, which has the aim of developing and implementing a national policy and lobbying for it in light of central government guidelines. On the other hand, the central government remains powerful because it determines any new physician position to be created, and must give permission for any major investment.

In England and Wales, responsibility at the subnational levels, the levels of the Regional and the Area health authorities, derives from formal delegation of authority downward. Parliament, through the 1973 Reorganization Act, gave the Secretary of State the duty to establish Regional and Area health authorities, and empowered him to direct these authorities to perform all the functions relating to the health services that he would specify. This pattern of delegation, and the relationships between the regional and local authorities and the central government, are much more formalized in England and Wales than in Sweden, following the principle that delegation downward should be matched by accountability upward. Moreover, the responsibilities of the subnational level seem to be limited to execution and administration, since the 1973 act states expressly that the secretary of state cannot delegate his principal duty of "securing the effective provision of the services."

In France the municipal level has no health care responsibilities. The responsibility of the regional level in France is mainly one of administrative coordination. With the recent tendency in France to decentralize, however, the regional level is slowly being involved in the preparation of the five-year plans.

In the Netherlands also, the responsibilities of the subnational level have been relatively minor up to now. The municipal level is involved in the enforcement of certain acts that relate more or less to health care, such as the Medical Practice Act and the Supply of Drugs Act. At the provincial level, until recently, the provincial councils of health have only had a coordinating and advisory function. A few years ago, however, they were given more important functions to fulfil in hospital planning. The 1974 Policy Proposal on the Structure of the Health Care System appears to call for much more power at the subnational level: under its recommendations, local and regional agencies would act in advisory and decision-making capacities, and the central government would be confined to outlining the general framework within which these powers could be exercised.

9 | Epilogue

The foregoing analysis of health resources development in five countries was intended to address a number of questions: why and how resources development took place; what forces and issues were operative; how interested parties participated and interacted; what role government played. Now, looking at health resources development in greater perspective, we can further reflect and speculate on some more general questions. Did some of the survey nations do better than others in resources development? If so, why? And to what extent is there a potential to learn from the experiences of other countries?

Was Anyone Doing Better?

Three dimensions are relevant for a cross-national evaluation of health resources development. One can look first at the volume of resources attained by the respective countries. Second, one can analyze the spatial distribution of the health resources in relation to the people they are to serve. Finally, one can consider the degree to which specialized and fragmented resources have been formally structured and integrated to function as a system capable of delivering comprehensive and integrated care to individual health care consumers.

The volume of health resources developed in each country can be compared by computing composite resource scores. In their international study on health care, Kohn and White constructed such resource scores for health manpower and hospital beds (Kohn and White 1976). Similar scores calculated for the survey nations provide a basis for comparing their respective social investments in basic health resources. The resource scores are based on the numbers of physicians, dentists, nurses, pharmacists, general hospital beds, and all other hospital beds per 10,000 population. In the composite score, the subscores for each professional group were multiplied by the average number of years of required training. The expense of training a physician is higher than that for a nurse or a dentist, so adjustment for this difference was made by applying the following weighting: seven for physicians, five for dentists, four for pharmacists, three for nurses. Since the development cost of a general hospital bed was considered equal to the production cost of a physician, a weighting of seven was also applied to general hospital beds. A weighting by four was used for other, less expensive hospital beds.

To some extent these weights are arbitrary, and the statistical data not totally accurate: such basic concepts as a general hospital bed and a nurse refer to different entities in the different survey nations (Blanpain 1977, p. 24). Nevertheless, although the scores obtained in this manner (see Table 3), represent very crude estimates, they do permit a ranking of the survey nations in their quantitative development efforts. Thus, the survey nations fall into three groups. Sweden is ahead, followed at some distance by a cluster formed by the Federal Republic of Germany, the Netherlands, and France; England and Wales trail far behind. High hospital figures and the above average development of dentists, physicians, nurses, and pharmacists make Sweden the leader in quantitative resources development. Paradoxically, Sweden's relatively high ratios of physicians and more particularly of dentists have not dispelled the ongoing Swedish concern about manpower shortages. Since 1948 Sweden has been seeking to correct its physician shortage, and until 1974 Sweden refrained from providing dental benefits under health insurance because of what was regarded as a shortage of dentists—despite the fact that the Swedish dentist ratio was more than double the average in the other countries.

At current growth rates, Swedish health manpower will rapidly exceed levels that other countries would consider as oversupply. The Swedes tend to be relaxed about this. The average number of working hours per week of health manpower is not well documented in the survey countries, but in Sweden, since the 1970 Seven Kronor Reform, the workweek for physicians has been a point of negotiation. Reduced working hours to forty per week could permit the system to absorb a substantial increase in manpower units (to remain at supply levels equivalent to these before the workweek reduction). An important factor in this Swedish lead in health resources has been the existence of the county councils. Because of their power to raise taxes and their nearly exclusive mandate in the health service field, they have been prime movers in resources development.

The comparatively low position of England and Wales in health resources development results primarily from low scores for hospitals, nurses, and dentists. The central government's rationing approach to hospital development and hospital-based nursing education is responsible for this state of affairs. Of course, this tradition of restraint might turn into an advantage as policies emerge that advocate limits on supply levels for reasons of cost-effectiveness. Should further evidence confirm these tendencies, England and Wales could find themselves in a better position than the other countries. The comparison of quantitative development scores reveals the interesting fact that although Sweden and England and Wales were the earliest among the survey nations to emphasize the supply side of their national health programs, they have ultimately followed very different courses of action, ending at opposite ends of the supply spectrum. Centralization in resource allocation and the low priority accorded to health services in competition with other national priorities put England and Wales at a disadvantage, while in Sweden decision-making has been more decentralized, with health matters virtually the single priority at the relevant decision-making level.

In the other countries, where the national health programs have concentrated on the benefits to be provided by a more or less independent provider community, the population covered has been increased by expanding reimbursement schemes. The impressive streams of money thus created have directly or indirectly supported capital investment and manpower development within the context of a "laissez-faire" attitude towards health facilities development, and within liberal and uncoordinated educational policies. The Federal Republic of Germany, the Netherlands, and to a lesser extent France have reached substantial resource levels in this way. Only recently have these countries started to affect the supply of resources directly, primarily with the intention of curbing this growth. Certification-of-need mechanisms have been introduced; special authorizations are required to build or renew facilities; subsidies for capital investment have become tied to planning criteria; limits on medical school enrollment have become standard procedure; ceilings on numbers of health care workers within the national health program are being considered.

Because of the strong bargaining position of the provider community, in particular doctors and to some extent hospitals, those countries that have relied on contributory health insurance to finance independent providers—France, the Federal Republic of Germany, and the Netherlands—have had more difficulty in determining adequate supply levels. In these countries the negotiating and advisory structures between the provider community and the government are heavily biased towards the problems of provider reimbursement. The national Ministry of Social Insurance traditionally has had a more dominant role than the Ministry of Health. Only recently have the ministries of health begun trying to ensure an adequate supply of health resources through planning. So far, however, these planning efforts have been hampered by underdevelopment of the administrative structures that are needed to relate the planning activities to the provider community, to the educational community, and to the populations to be served. In contrast, England and Wales, and more particularly Sweden, are more advanced, having health resource planning and allocation structures that permit goal-oriented planning cycles, which are attuned to the broader framework of socioeconomic planning, on the one hand, and to the institutionalized developers of health resources, on the other.

Nevertheless, all five countries are confronted with the problem of how to define adequate national supply levels. By and large, the survey nations still rely mainly on an advisory machinery, manned largely by representatives of the provider community, to determine criteria and standards for the supply of health resources. Occasionally this advisory process is short-circuited by government decision—for example, in the Netherlands, where State Secretary Hendriks abruptly mandated a norm of four general hospital beds per thousand population in 1976. All countries face the problem of developing scientifically based requirements for health resources. The limited attention given to epidemiology is a handicap in this respect. Among the survey nations, England and Wales seem to have realized this need earlier than the other countries, and have taken initiative to correct the situation.

With respect to the distribution of resources, the countries fall into two groups. Sweden and England and Wales began to consider geographic distribution much earlier than the other countries did. Regionalization of hospital care and measures to affect maldistribution of physicians were introduced before World War II in Sweden, and in 1948 in England and Wales. Nevertheless, discrepancies continue to exist. In Sweden in 1972, physician density per thousand inhabitants was still limited to 0.9 in several counties versus 3.0 in Uppsala County. The other countries left the distribution of resources more or less to market forces until the late sixties, when they began to discuss possible means of government regulation to diminish the ranges between underserved and overserved areas. Determining such areas to begin with presents methodological problems, since the necessary data-resources are usually underdeveloped and it is often difficult to reach agreement whether a given area is underserved or overserved. The burden of proof is sometimes placed on the government, which in turn depends on information from the providers to justify its position. The complicated approaches used to redistribute resources, including financial incentives such as bonuses for underserved areas or liquidation funds for overserved areas, are still too tentative to permit any assessment of their workability. The future will show whether they can affect maldistribution. There are also differences in the degree to which the survey countries have managed to structure their resources into a health care system in which the components are formally articulated, interdependent, and responsive to the full spectrum of community needs. England and Wales, particularly since the 1973 Reorganization of the National Health Service, have progressed furthest in this respect, followed by Sweden, which has gradually but continuously moved towards meshing the different components—such as hospital care, ambulatory care, preventive care, extended care, and social welfare—into an integrated system. Both these countries have also managed to bring their administrative geographic subdivisions in line with the geographic subdivisions of the health care system.

Of the three other countries, only the Netherlands has explicitly formulated a more structured and interrelated health care system adjusted to an administrative reorganization of its territory. But the Dutch still face the formidable task of implementing these plans. Meanwhile, France and the Federal Republic of Germany have not yet finished discussing the issue—the inadequate coordination and integration of different types of health care in the same geographic area; an inadequate flow of information, patients and staff among different tiers in the health services; and the ironic imbalance in emphasis in favor of uncommon health problems and to the detriment of more common problems.

Beyond these assessments, it is difficult to answer definitively the question of whether one country did better than another in terms of volume of health resources, spatial distribution of resources, and structuring of resources. The ultimate validation of efforts in resource development should be the health status of the population, which is, after all, the overall purpose of health resources development. Countries could be compared in relation to statistics like the degree of survival, levels of somatic or nonsomatic morbidity, and disability. But a major difficulty in the comparative evaluation of the health status of populations is the lack of generally accepted and suitable indicators. While mortality data are commonly used as indicators for death or survival, indicators for attributes such as morbidity, disability, distress, and so on, have not yet been internationally agreed upon. Composite health status indices are still in the early stages of development and include so many value judgments that they would not be generally applicable even if the needed data were available (Greene 1976, p. 39). Within this set of constraints, and using four current indicators—male life expectancy at the age of one year, maternal mortality, perinatal mortality, and infant mortality—the five countries present for 1971 a very consistent pattern: Sweden is best on all five indicators, followed by the Netherlands, which ranks second on all indicators; England and Wales is third on four of the indicators; France is third on the infant mortality indicator and fourth on the rest; West Germany trails on every indicator (Table 4). It must be noted that this type of assessment is based on the assumption that the health status of the population results primarily from health services, so that health status can be correlated with factors such as the volume, distribution, and organization of health resources. In fact, this assumption itself is questionable and is being challenged by some who claim that health services have only a marginal effect on life expectancy. Genetics, nutrition, environmental sanitation, life style, and accident prevention are considered more important to health than health services are (Dubos 1959) (McKeown 1976). The high ranking of Sweden and the Netherlands in health status indicators is undoubtedly due to factors outside the health services, so that this ranking provides no answers to the question of how resources should be developed. This is obviously a fertile field for in-depth investigation. Already Canada has begun to commit itself, despite some ongoing controversy, to the view that health services are not the sole guarantee of health, and that health policy should be redirected to deemphasize health resources (Lalonde 1974).

Improving the Efficiency of Learning

Throughout the development of their national health programs, the survey countries sought to learn from the experience of other countries. This interest in a neighbor's solutions was more intense at times when important changes were being considered. For example, in both England and Wales and in France the introduction of compulsory sickness insurance was accompanied by study and controversy about the system in operation in Germany.

Immediately after World War II, there was much ferment over national health programs in most European countries. Existing compulsory health insurance was substantially extended in coverage and benefits, or a national health service was introduced, as in England and Wales. A number of governments that had been in exile in London were exposed to the preparations for the National Health Service. After the war, therefore, the British model was studied and discussed in the Netherlands and Sweden.

In the 1950s, supranational organizations like the World Health Organization, the International Labor Office, the Office of Economic Development and Cooperation, and the Council of Europe started to promote cross-national studies of health care delivery, health insurance, health facilities, health manpower, health economics, and health planning. The academic establishment showed a growing interest, with increasing attempts to reach beyond mere description toward systematic comparative studies. So far, however, most of these attempts have examined only limited aspects of the health care system. Availability, reliability, and comparability of data still present serious problems that should be addressed in a more focused way.

The beginning of the seventies has been characterized by what some have called an "epidemic" of national health program reforms. Indeed, not only the survey nations, but most other countries in Europe and North America have witnessed an unprecedented cascade of legislative action and government regulation to reshape the health care system. The result is a new impetus for cross-national studies, and new supranational agencies are sponsoring and promoting such studies. For example, the European Economic Community has recently begun to commission comparative health care studies. Even NATO, through its Committee on the Challenges for Modern Society, has embarked on international health care research. Some of these studies are repetitive, indicating both urgency and a lack of consultation between the sponsors. At the time of the study leading to this publication, five international inventories of national studies of health costs were being conducted simultaneously in Europe, commissioned respectively by the World Health Organization, the International Labor Office, the European Economic Community, the Sandoz Institute for Health Services Research, and an American management consultant firm.

Another indication of the sharpened interest in other countries' experiences is that national consultative bodies established to review the problems of their national health programs are explicitly looking at systems abroad. The royal commissioner appointed in Belgium in March 1975 to present proposals for reorganization of the national health program, in his report submitted in February 1976, refers continually to other countries, particularly in Europe (Petit 1976). Likewise, the Royal Commission on the National Health Service, created in Great Britain in 1976, "to consider in the interests both of the patients and of those who work in the National Health Service the best use and management of the financial and manpower resources" (Royal Commission 1976), began to examine other nations early in its investigations. The Nuffield Provincial Hospitals Trust was asked to organize a private seminar in April 1977 with selected health officials and scholars from continental Europe and the United States. The commission hopes to learn how these countries are coping with problems of availability and access of services, cost-containment and cost-control, freedom of initiative, provider negotiations, and the relation between education and service.

Such initiatives and studies reflect the widespread feeling that the recent climax in national decision-making, legislation, and regulation has overshot the mark, resulting in a deadlock. Some recent plans have either proved to be overambitious, given existing information and management resources, or have turned out to be less acceptable to the provider community or the public than had been anticipated. Despite government legislation, there is a climate of "muddling through"; the reaction is an increased awareness of the need to develop better information resources and more mission-oriented health services research. Thus, there is a growing interest in finding out how other countries are currently approaching similar problems during the stage of policy discussion and formulation. An "intelligence dimension" to monitor the first indications of new developments is being added to the scholarly quest to understand how other systems function.

The health services research community is confronted with a double challenge. In the first place, particular structures, methodologies, and techniques, particularly in respect to planning and evaluation, need to be made available in advance of policy developments that will require them for successful implementation. Secondly, a more in-depth analysis and assessment of policy development is necessary, at the time policy is being formulated, not only to contribute to national policy-making, but also to provide a more efficient way to share knowledge at the international level, at a time when such sharing is still relevant to policies or problems under consideration. These challenges are highly interrelated, and depend on the capacity to monitor policy development.

The comparative study of health care could be supplemented in a number of ways to strengthen this policy-monitoring capacity. An intelligence network could be established in which selected research centers would be responsible at an early stage for communicating important policy developments in their own country to comparable centers abroad, in order to provide, within a reasonable time, a follow-up analysis of these developments. Such a network would, of course, require formal relationships between the research centers and those agencies, either governmental or nongovernmental, responsible for discussing and formulating health care policy. Developments such as Plan-line, currently being worked out in the U.S. Department of Health, Education, and Welfare, eventually will provide updated on-line communication of health planning publications, including documents with limited circulation, through an information network comparable to the world wide Medical Literature Analysis and Retrieval System (MEDLARS).

Some twenty nations, under sponsorship of the World Health Organization and the U.S. Department of Health, Education, and Welfare, are urging health services researchers to focus on case studies of the structure, processes, and methods of health planning. A serious and focused effort to make national health resources data more detailed, reliable, and comparable, in particular in the field of manpower, is important to comparative health studies. The World Health Organization's efforts could perhaps be supplemented by a lead agency, such as the U.S. National Center for Health Statistics, which has a remarkable record of providing international and bilateral assistance to the national vital statistics services of other countries. A similar commitment to the development of health resources statistics would undoubtedly improve the quality of needed international health care studies.

Finally, there are few forums through which cross-national health care experience can rapidly be made available. The exchange of ideas requires modes that are quicker than publications and that allow more give-and-take. Agencies like the Nuffield Provincial Hospitals Trust in London and the Fogarty International Center at the National Institutes of Health in Bethesda have been the forerunners in organizing face-to-face exchanges on health care problems in different countries. Let us hope that others will be inspired by their example.

TABLES

BIBLIOGRAPHY

INDEX

Table 1. Statistics for 1971

	Sweden	The Netherlands	England and Wales	France	Federal Republic of Germany	USA
Vital statistics						
Population (millions)	8.10	13.19	48.85	51.25	61.29	207.05
Population per sq. km	18	323	323	94	247	22
Population in rural areas [a] (%)	20.4	19	21.6	30.1	18.8	25.9
Life expectancy at age One						
Males	72	71	69.6	69.1	68.3	67.9
Females	77.3	76.7	75.7	76.7	74.4	75.2
Population 65 and older (%)	13.9	10.2	13.4	13.5	13.4	9.9
Perinatal mortality per 1,000 live births	15.7	17.8	22.5	22.8	25.6	27.1 [b]
Infant mortality per 1,000 live births	11.1	12.1	17.3	16	22.8	18.5
Maternal mortality per 100,000 live births	7.9	12.1	16.9	22.2	50.4	20.5
Health resources						
All hospital beds per 1,000 pop.	16.57	11.74 [d]	9.24	10.39	11.26	7.51
General hospital beds per 1,000 pop.	6.94	5.36	4.07	6.05	6.68	4.67
Psychiatric beds per 1,000 pop.	6.21	3.54	3.59	2.30	1.87	2.77 [a]
Physicians per 10,000 pop.	13.9	13.2	12.7	13.9	17.8	15.4
Dentists per 10,000 pop.	8.2	2.6	2.7	4.1	5.1	5.1

Qualified nurses per 10,000 pop.[a]	40.7	44.8[c]	30.7	26.6	23.1	35.3
Pharmacists per 10,000 pop.	4.0	0.8	2.8	5.2	5.6[a]	6.3
Hospital ownership (% of total beds)						
Government	99	25[b]	98[e]	65[b]	54.2[a]	33.4
Private nonprofit		75[b]		9[b]	43.6[a]	61.2
Private profit	1		2[e]	26[b]	2.1[a]	5.5
Health care expenditure						
GNP spent on health services (%)	7.0	7.3[d]	4.9[e]	5.6	5.7[c]	7.5
Increases in percentage of GNP spent on health services between 1960 and 1969	2.9	1.4	0.7[e]	1.4	1.2	1.5
Annual health expenditure per person (US $)[c]	234	116	93[e]	140	154	298
Resource utilization						
Admissions to general hospitals per 10,000 population[a]	1495	967	1015	720[f]	1125	1480
Admissions per bed per annum in general hospitals	22	17.6	25.1	15.9[f]	17.3	31

Sources: R. Maxwell, *Health care: the growing dilemma* (New York: McKinsey, 1975); *International health costs and expenditures* (Washington, D.C.: U.S. Dept. of Health, Education, and Welfare, 1976). [a] 1970 [b] 1968 [c] 1969 [d] 1972 [e] UK [f] Public only

Table 2. Benefits at the start of public health insurance

Nation	Date of enactment	Start of program	Benefits				
			Medical			Dental Care	Prescr. Drugs
			GP	Spec.	Hosp.		
Germany	June 15, 1883	December 1, 1884	x	x	x		x
England and Wales	December 16, 1911	January 1, 1913	x	x			x
France	April 30, 1930	July 1, 1930	x	x	x		x
The Netherlands	August 1, 1941	November 1, 1941	x	x	x	x	
Sweden	January 3, 1947	January 1, 1955	x	x	x		x

Table 3. Health manpower, hospital beds, and composite resource scores per 10,000 inhabitants in the survey nations in 1971

	Sweden	Netherlands	England and Wales	France	Federal Republic of Germany	Weight	Average
Physicians	13.9	13.2	12.7	13.9	17.8	7	14.3
Nurses	40.7	44.8	30.7	26.6	23.1	3	33.18
Dentists	8.2	2.6	2.7	4.1	5.1	5	4.54
Pharmacists	4.0	0.8	2.8	5.2	5.6	4	3.68
Manpower score	276.4	243.0	205.7	218.4	241.8	—	237.06
Manpower rank	1	2	5	4	3	—	—
General beds	69.4	53.6	40.7	60.5	66.8	7	58.2
Other beds	96.3	63.8	51.7	43.4	45.8	4	60.2
Bed score	871.0	630.4	491.7	597.1	650.8	—	648.2
Bed rank	1	3	5	4	2	—	—
Total score	1147.4	873.4	697.4	815.5	892.6	—	885.26
Rank	1	3	5	4	2	—	—

Source: See Table 1.

Table 4. Ranking of survey nations by selected health indicators in 1971

Nation	Life expectancy: males at age one	Perinatal mortality	Infant mortality	Maternal mortality
Sweden	1	1	1	1
The Netherlands	2	2	2	2
England and Wales	3	3	4	3
France	4	4	3	4
Federal Republic of Germany	5	5	5	5

Source: See Table 1.

Bibliography

Abel-Smith, B. 1964. *The hospitals 1800–1948*. London: Heinemann.

Adam, W. 1973. *Modernes Krankenhaus*. Vol. 18. Cologne, Berlin: Grote'sche Verlagsbuchhandlung K G.

Albrecht, R. G. 1975. Uber den Ausgangspunkt der Beziehungen der Ärzte zu den Krankenkassen. *Zentralblatt für Sozialsicherung, Socialhilfe und Versorgung* 5–6:140–80.

Alva Myrdal report: towards equality. Stockholm: Bokförlaget, Prisma.

American Academy of Arts and Sciences. 1977. Doing better and feeling worse: health in the United States. In *Proceedings of the American Academy of Arts and Sciences* 1.

American Hospital Association. 1974. *Analysis of national health insurance proposals*. Chicago.

Anderson, N., and L. Robins. 1976. Observations on potential contributions of health planning. *International Journal of Health Services* 6:651–66.

Anderson, O. W. 1971. Styles of planning services: the United States, Sweden and England. *International Journal of Health Services* 1:106–21.

———. 1972. *Health care: can there be equity?* New York: John Wiley.

Andriessen, L. B. 1966. De algemene wet zware geneeskundige risico's. *Ons Ziekenhuis* 28:70–76.

Approbationsordnung für Ärzte. 1970. *Bundesgesetzblatt* 1970:1458.

Aujaleu, E. La planification hospitalière en France.

Austin, C., J. Ball, and D. Clark. 1975. Education for health administration: a statistical profile. In *Education for health administration*, pp. 71–143. Ann Arbor: Health Administration Press.

Batistella, R. 1971. National health insurance: an examination of leading proposals in the light of contemporary policy issues. *Inquiry* 8:20–36.

Bierman, P., E. Connors, E. Flook, R. Huntley, T. McCarthy, and P. Sanazaro. 1968. Health services research in Britain. *Milbank Memorial Fund Quarterly* 46:1.

Blanpain, J. 1968. The development of health sciences centers in an international perspective. In *Proceedings of the national seminar on planning and construction of health sciences centers,* pp. 87–100. Ottawa: Department of Health and Welfare.

———. 1973. E.E.C.: the founding six. In *Health services prospects: an international survey,* pp. 37–54. London: *The Lancet* and the Nuffield Provincial Hospitals Trust.

———. 1975. De gezondheidszorg en de E.E.G.: een uitdaging. *Acta Hospitalia* 15:267–78.

———. 1975. Rol en funktie van het ziekenhuis in de gezondheidszorg van de E.E.G. landen. *Leiding* 28:171–85.

———. 1977. The role and function of the hospital in the E.E.C. health care systems. In *Health services systems in the European Economic Community,* pp. 84–99. Washington, D.C.: Department of Health, Education, and Welfare.

Blanpain, J., and L. Delesie. 1976. *Community health investment.* London: Oxford University Press for the Nuffield Provincial Hospitals Trust.

Boer, E. P. D. 1966. Een beschouwing over de algemene verzekering zware geneeskundige risico's. *Tijdschrift voor Sociale Geneeskunde* 44:498–502.

Brand, J. L. 1965. *Doctors and the state.* Baltimore: Johns Hopkins University Press.

Bridgman, R. F. 1971. Medical care under social security in France. *International Journal of Health Services* 1:331–41.

Britain 1974, an official handbook. London: HMSO.

British Medical Association. 1970. Report of council to special representative meeting. *British Medical Journal Supplement* 3403:23–31.

British Medical Association. 1973. Letter to the profession: progress report. *British Medical Journal Supplement* 3540:29.

Brown, R. G. S. 1973. *The changing national health service.* London: Routledge and Kegan Paul.

Bruce, M. 1974. *The coming of the welfare state.* 4th ed. London: Batsford.

Bundesministerium für Bildung und Wissenschaft. 1972. *Forschungsbericht des Bundesministerium für Bildung und Wissenschaft.* Bonn.

Bundesministerium für Jugend, Familie und Gesundheit. 1975. Bericht der Bundesregierung über die Auswerkingen des Krankenhausfinanzierungsgesetzes. *Druchsache* 7:4530.

———. 1975. Entwurf eines Gesetzes zur Weiterentwicklung des Kassenarztrechts und zur Änderung der Krankensicherung der Rentner. *Druchsache* 7:3336.

Burg, C. 1973. The organization and support of biomedical research in France. In *Medical research systems in Europe,* pp. 67–76. Amsterdam: Elsevier, Excerpta Medica.

Central Bureau of Statistics. 1973. *Diagnose Statistiek Ziekenhuizen.* The Hague: Staatsuitgeverij.

Central Office of Information. 1973. *Health Services in Britain.* London: HMSO.

Charney, S. D. 1969. *Doctors: surplus or shortage.* New Haven: Yale University.

Chesney, A. M. 1958. *Johns Hopkins Hospital and the Johns Hopkins University School of Medicine.* Baltimore: Johns Hopkins University Press.

Chester, T. E. *The reorganization of the N.H.S. in perspective.*
———. 1969. Organization for the operation of the national health service. In *The British National Health Service,* pp. 19–34. Chicago: ACHA.
———. 1970. Educational programmes for hospital administrators in the U.K. and the U.S.A. *Acta Hospitalia* 10:343–57.
———. 1975. The reorganization of the N.H.S., blue print and reality. *World Hospitals* 11:10–16.
Cochrane, A. 1972. *Effectiveness and efficiency.* London: Oxford University Press for the Nuffield Provincial Hospitals Trust.
Cohen, R. 1971. The department's role in research and development. In *Portfolio for Health 1,* pp. 1–22. London: Oxford University Press for the Nuffield Provincial Hospitals Trust.
College voor Ziekenhuisvoorzieningen. 1975. *Advies wet ziekenhuisvoorzieningen.* Utrecht.
Comet, P. 1965. *L'hôpital public.* Paris: Berger.
Commission de la santé et de l'assurance maladie pour le septième plan, la. 1976. Rapport général. *L'Hôpital à Paris* 32:113–59.
Confédération des Syndicats médicaux français. 1976. *Médecin de France,* April.
Courquet, J. 1971. *L'hôpital aujourd'hui et demain.* Paris: Seuil.
Crossman, R. 1970. *The future structure of the N.H.S.: green paper 2.* London: HMSO.
Davis, K. 1976. *Excerpta Medica travel award 1975.* Amsterdam: Excerpta Medica Foundation.
De Bono, E. 1976. *Practical thinking.* London: Penguin.
Decker, B., and P. Bonner. 1973. *P.S.R.O.: organization for regional peer review.* Cambridge, Mass.: Ballinger.
Décret 58-1202 relatif aux hôpitaux et hospices publics. 1958. *Journal Officiel* 12.
De Groot, M. J. W. 1972. Computer en gezondheidsstatistiek. In *Computer en medische zorg,* pp. 135–55. Leiden: Stafleu.
Department of Health, Education, and Welfare (U.S.). 1976. *Health Services News 4.* Washington, D.C.: Health Resources Administration.
Department of Health and Social Security (U.K.). 1972a. *Management arrangements for the reorganized national health service.* London: HMSO.
———. 1972b. *Report of the working party on medical administrators.* London: HMSO.
———. 1974. *Annual report 1973.* London: HMSO.
———. 1976. *Priorities for health and personal social services in England.* London: HMSO.
Deutsche Krankenhaus Gesellschaft. 1970. Entwurf eines Gesetzes der Geschäftsführung der Deutschen Krankenhausgesellschaft über die wirtschaftliche Sicherung der Krankenhäuser und über die Regelung der Krankenhauspflegesätze vom August 4, 1970. *Das Krankenhaus* 62:327–32.
———. 1971. Stellungnahme der Deutsche Krankenhaus Gesellschaft. *Das Krankenhaus* 63:193–200.

Dolman, D. 1968. Uit het parlement. *Tijdschrift voor Sociale Geneeskunde* 46:65.

Dorsey, J. 1975. The health maintenance organization act of 1973 (P.L.93–222) and prepaid group practice plans. *Medical Care* 13:1–19.

Dubos, R. 1959. *Mirage of Health.* New York: Harper & Row.

Duchesne, E. 1897. *Contribution à l'étude de la concurrence vitale chez les microorganismes. Antagonisme entre les moisisures et les microbes.* Lyon.

Dupeyroux, J. J. 1975. *Droit de la sécurité sociale.* Paris: Dalloz.

Eckstein, H. 1958. *The English health service.* Cambridge, Mass.: Harvard University Press.

Ecole Nationale de la Santé Publique. 1974. *L'organisation sanitaire française.* Rennes.

Eichhorn, S. 1973. The Federal Republic of Germany. In *Health services prospects: an international survey,* pp. 81–98. London: *The Lancet* and the Nuffield Provincial Hospitals Trust.

Engel, A. 1968. Planning and spontaneity in the development of the Swedish health system. In *The 1968 Michael M. Davis Lecture,* pp. 1–22. Chicago: Center for Health Administration Studies.

———. 1971. Regional planning. In *The Swedish health services system,* pp. 63–80. Chicago: ACHA.

English, M. L. 1976. Budgeting for national health expenditure: the British system. *World Hospitals* 12:164–70.

Excerpta Medica. 1973. *Medical research systems in Europe.* Amsterdam: Elsevier.

Federation of Swedish county councils. 1971. *Swedish medical care in the 1980's: ways and means.* Stockholm.

Festen, H. 1974. *125 jaar geneeskunst en Maatschappij.* Utrecht: KNMG.

Fleischhauer, K. 1973. Medical education, care and research in the Federal Republic of Germany. In *Medical research systems in Europe,* pp. 89–102. Amsterdam: Elsevier, Excerpta Medica.

Fleming, A. 1929. On the antibacterial actions of cultures of a penicillium with special reference to their use in the isolation of B. Influenza. *British Journal of Experimental Pathology.*

Foot, M. 1973. *Aneurin Bevan 1945–1960.* London: Davis-Poynter.

Forsyth, G., and R. Logan. 1960. *The demand for medical care: a study of the case load in the Barrow and Furness group of hospitals.* London: Oxford University Press for the Nuffield Provincial Hospitals Trust.

Fraser, D. 1973. *The evolution of the British welfare state.* London: Macmillan.

Galant, H. 1955. *Histoire politique de la sécurité sociale française.* Paris: Cahiers de la Fondation des sciences politiques.

Gatherer, A. 1971. Community medicine: quo vadis? In *Challenges for Change,* pp. 95–128. London: Oxford University Press for the Nuffield Provincial Hospitals Trust.

Gerfeldt, E. 1959. *Das Krankenhaus und seine Betriebsführung.* Stuttgart: Gustave Fisher.

Gesetzliche Krankenversicherung. 1883. *Reichtsgesetzblatt* 1883:73–104.

Gesetz zur Ordnung der Krankenpflege. 1938. *Reichsgesetzblatt* 1938:1309.

Gesetz über Ausübung des Berufes des Krankenschwester, des Krankenpflegers und der Kinderkrankenschwester. 1957. *Bundesgesetzblatt* 1957:716.

Gesetz zur wirtschaftlichen Sicherung der Krankenhäuser und zur Regelung der Krankenhauspflegesätze. 1972. *Bundesgesetzblatt* 1972:1009.

Gesetz zur Weiterentwicklung der Kassenarztrechts. 1976. *Bundesgesetzblatt* 1976:3871–77.

Godber, G. 1975. *The health services: past, present and future.* London: Athlone Press.

Greene, R. 1976. Assuring quality in medical care. Cambridge, Mass.: Ballinger.

Groot, L., H. Van Aert, W. Van Montfort, and L. Verheyen. 1974. 1975. *Basisonderzoek kostenstructuur ziekenhuizen.* Utrecht: Nationaal Ziekenhuisinstituut.

Guiheneuf, L. 1967. *Financiële kontekst van de groepspraktijk in Frankrijk.* Brussels: Studie- en adviesbureau groepspraktijk voor huisartsen.

Gunn, L., and R. Mair. 1971. Staffing the national health service. In *Challenges for change,* pp. 263–95. London: Oxford University Press for the Nuffield Provincial Hospitals Trust.

Hall, P. 1974. Current status of the Karolinska Hospital computer system. In *Hospital computers system,* pp. 546–97. New York: John Wiley.

Hatzfeld, H. 1963. *Le grand tournant de la médecine liberale.* Paris: les éditions ouvrières.

———. 1971. *Du paupérisme à la sécurité sociale.* Paris: Colin.

Health services act, The. 1976. *The Hospital and Health Services Review* 73:72–74.

Hebammergesetz. 1938. *Reichsgesetzblatt* 1938:1893.

Henry, P. 1930. Notice sous la loi du 30 avril 1930. *Annuaire de législation française* 1930:99–104.

Herder-Dorneich, P. 1970. *Honorar Reform und Krankenhaussanierung.* Cologne: Erich Schmidt.

Hogarth, J. 1963. *The payment of the general practitioner.* Oxford: Pergamon.

Högberg, G. 1971. The development and status of hospital administration. In *The Swedish health services system,* pp. 81–100. Chicago: ACHA.

Honigsbaum, F. 1970. *The struggle for the ministry of health 1914–1919.* London: Bell.

Hulten, F. F. H., J. Van der Gaag, and B. M. S. van Praag. 1975. *Het ziekenhuis in de gezondheidszorg.* Leiden: Stenfert-Kroese.

Huysmans, F. 1973. *Gezondheidszorg in Nederland.* Nijmegen: SUN.

Iba Zizen, M. 1973. La réforme hospitalière et les décrets d'application. *Hospitalisation Privée* 1973:169–77.

Illich, I. 1975. *Medical nemesis: the expropriation of health.* London: Colder and Boyars.

Inspection générale des affaires sociales. 1972. Rapport annuel 1971. *La Revue Hospitalière de France* 36:1031–1157.

International association of social security. 1972. *The general causes of the increase in sickness insurance expenditure in Sweden 1955–1970.* Stockholm: Riksförsäkringsverket.

Internationale vereniging voor sociale zekerheid. 1959. *Ontwikkeling en tendenties van de sociale zekerheid in Nederland.* Geneva.

Jambu-Merlin, R. 1970. *La sécurité sociale.* Paris: Colin.

Jonsson, E. 1971. *The organization and financing of medical services in Sweden.* Stockholm: SPRI.

Joseph, K. 1972. *National health service reorganization: England (white paper).* London: HMSO.

Klarman, H. 1963. *Hospital care in New York City.* New York: Columbia University Press.

Kohn, R., and K. White. 1976. *Health care: an international study.* London: Oxford University Press.

Koninklijke Nederlandse Maatschappij Geneeskunst. 1946. Organisatieplan van de volksgezondheid. *Medisch Contact* 1:12–29.

———. 1974. Structuurnota gezondheidszorg. Memorandum K.N.M.G. *Medisch Contact* 29:1377–83.

———. 1976. Uitbreiding ziekenhuisfunkties aan onjuiste voorwaarden gebonden. *Medisch Contact* 31:1494.

Kulp, B., and W. Schreiber. 1971. *Soziale Sicherheit.* Cologne, Berlin: Kiepenheuer and Witsch.

Lalonde, M. 1974. *A new perspective on the health of Canadians.* Ottawa: Ministry of Health and Welfare.

Landelijke Huisartsen Vereniging. 1975. *Blauwdruk Beleid L. H. V.* Utrecht: KNMG.

Landelijk Informatiesysteem Ziekenfondsen. 1974. *Jaarboek 1973.* Utrecht: GOZ.

Landelijke Specialisten Vereniging. 1976. *Intercollegiale toetsing in algemene ziekenhuizen.* Utrecht.

Landstingsförbundet and Socialstyrelsen. 1975. *Landstingens Planer 1974–1980 (LKELP 75).* Stockholm.

Ledeboer, L. V. 1966. *De Ziekenfondsverzekering in Nederland.* 2nd ed. Amstelveen: De Ziekenfondsraad.

Levy, H. 1944. *National health insurance: a critical study.* Cambridge: Cambridge University Press.

Lindberg, G. 1949. *Den Svenska Sjukkasserörelsen Historica.* Lund.

Lindgren, S. 1967. Yesterday, today, tomorrow: a close-up of the regional plan. In *Regional hospital planning: in honour of A. Engel.* Stockholm: National Board of Health.

———. 1973. Sweden. In *Health services prospects: an international survey,* pp. 99–124. London: *The Lancet* and the Nuffield Provincial Hospitals Trust.

Lindsey, A. 1962. *Socialized medicine in England and Wales.* Chapel Hill: University of North Carolina Press.

Loi du 5 avril 1928 sur les assurances sociales. *Annuaire de législation française* 1928:170–232.

Loi du 30 avril 1930 modifiant et completant la loi du 5 avril 1928 sur les assurances sociales. *Annuaire de législation française* 1930:99–164.

Loi du 31 décembre 1970 portant Réforme Hospitalière. *Journal Officiel,* January 3, 1971:67.

Lynch, M. J., and S. S. Raphael. 1963. *Medicine and the State.* Springfield, Illinois: Charles C. Thomas.

Mandeville, L. 1974. L'assurance: maladie et l'hospitalisation. *Revue de droit sanitaire et sociale* 1974:37–38.

Manevy, J. V. 1976. Médecine: la fin du monopole de Paris. *L'Express* 1279:67–69.

Mannoury, J. 1966. Ziekenfondsenbesluit 25 jaar. *Sociaal Maandblad Arbeid* 1966:683–84.

Maxwell, R. 1975. *Health care: the growing dilemma.* New York: McKinsey.

———. 1976. International health costs and expenditures. In *International health costs and expenditures,* pp. 3–22. Washington, D.C.: Department of Health, Education, and Welfare.

McLachlan, G. 1971. 1973. *Portfolio for health 1, 2.* London: Oxford University Press for the Nuffield Provincial Hospitals Trust.

———. 1974. *Positions and directions in health services research.* London: Oxford University Press for the Nuffield Provincial Hospitals Trust.

———. 1976. *A question of quality.* London: Oxford University Press for the Nuffield Provincial Hospitals Trust.

McKeown, T. 1965. *A balanced teaching hospital.* London: Oxford University Press for the Nuffield Provincial Hospitals Trust.

———. 1976. *The role of medicine: dreams, mirage or nemesis.* London: Oxford University Press for the Nuffield Provincial Hospitals Trust.

Ministère de la Santé Publique. 1970. *Projet de loi portant réforme hospitalière: Exposé des motifs.*

Ministère de la Santé Publique. 1973. L'hospitalisation publique en France. *Revue française des affaires sociales* 1973 (special number).

Ministerie van Cultuur, Recreatie en Maatschappelijk Werk, and Ministerie van Volksgezondheid en Milieuhygiëne. 1974. *Voorlopige stimuleringsregeling gezondheidscentra.* Rijswijk, July 8. Leidschendam, July 3.

Ministerie van Financiën. 1976. *Rijksbegroting 1976: XVII. Memorie van Toelichting. Openbare bespreking.* The Hague: Tweede Kamer (1975–1976).

Ministerie van Sociale Zaken en Volksgezondheid. 1966. *Volksgezondheidsnota.* The Hague: Staatsuitgeverij.

Ministerie van Volksgezondheid en Milieuhygiëne. 1974. *Concept ontwerp van wet tot wijziging van de wet Ziekenhuisvoorzieningen en Memorie van Toelichting.* Leidschendam.

Ministerie van Volksgezondheid en Milieuhygiëne. 1975a (September). *Nota A.S.G.29.* Leidschendam.

Ministerie van Volksgezondheid en Milieuhygiëne. 1975b (October). *Brieven nr.47.500; 48.762; 48.765; 48.966; 49.010.* Leidschendam.

Ministerie van Volksgezondheid en Milieuhygiëne. 1976. *Regelen ter bevordering van een doelmatig stelsel van voorzieningen voor gezondheidszorg.* The Hague: Tweede Kamer (1976–1977. 14.181).

Ministerie van Volksgezondheid en Milieuhygiëne. 1976. *Regelen m.b.t. de tarieven van organen voor gezondheidszorg.* The Hague: Tweede Kamer (1976–1977. 14.182).

Minister van Sociale Zaken en Volksgezondheid. 1966. Antwoord van de Minister van Sociale Zaken en Volksgezondheid aan de leden van de Tweede Kamer Commissie—Uittreksel. *Ons Ziekenhuis* 28:284–86.

Ministry of Health. *National Health Services Notes.* London.

Ministry of Health. 1956. *Report of the Committee on Inquiry into the Cost of the N.H.S. (the Guillebaud Report).* London: HMSO.

Ministry of Health. 1962. *A hospital plan for England and Wales.* London: HMSO.

Ministry of Health. 1966. *Report of the Committees on Senior Nursing Structure (the Salmon Report).* London: HMSO.

Ministry of Public Health and Environmental Hygiene, and Central Bureau of Statistics. 1974. *Compendium of health statistics of the Netherlands 1974.* The Hague: Staatsuitgeverij.

Monde, Le. March 17, 1976. *Les doyens des facultés de médecine recommandent une présélection au niveau du baccalauréat.*

——. April 28, 1976(a). *Les doyens des facultés ont continué leurs travaux de réflexion sur les études médicales.*

——. April 28, 1976(b). *Renforcer la sélection.*

——. May 26, 1976. *Les doyens des facultés de médecine n'ont pu se mettre d'accord sur le problème de l'accès aux spécialités.*

Naschold, F. 1967. *Kassenärzte und Krankenversicherungsreform.* Freiburg im Breisgau: Rombach.

National Board of Health and Welfare. 1969. *Program of principles for open medical care.* Stockholm: Nordiska Bokhandeln.

National Health Service Act, The. 1946. *Current Law Statutes Annotated* 1946: Chapter 81.

National Health Service Reorganization Act, The. 1973. *Current Law Statutes Annotated* 1973: Chapter 32.

National Insurance Act, The. 1911. *Current Law Statutes Annotated* 1911: Chapter 55.

National Insurance Act, The. 1962. Stockholm: Ministry of Health and Social Affairs.

Nationaal Ziekenhuis Instituut. 1974. *Financiële statistiek 1973. Verpleeghuizen, ziekenhuizen.* Utrecht.

Nationale Ziekenhuisraad. 1974. Bestuur geeft commentaar op de Structuurnota Gezondheidszorg. *Het Ziekenhuis* 4:524–26.

——. 1975. *Kommentaar koncept ontwerp van wet tòt wijziging van de wet ziekenhuisvoorzieningen.* Utrecht.

——. 1976. Voorwaarden uitbreiding ziekenhuisfuncties. *Medisch Contact* 31:1333.

Navarro, V. 1972. *National and regional health planning in Sweden.* Washington, D.C.: Department of Health, Education, and Welfare.

Neufassung der Bundesärzte Ordnung. 1970. *Bundesgesetzblatt* 1970:237.

Notverordnung. 1923. *Reichsgesetzblatt* 1923:1051.

Ordonnance 58-1198 portant réforme de la législation hospitalière. 1958. *Journal Officiel,* December 12, 1958.

Ordonnance 58-1199 relative à la coordination des établissements de soins comportant hospitalisation. 1958. *Journal Officiel,* December 12, 1958.

Ordonnance 58-1373 relative à la création de centres hospitaliers et universitaires, à la réforme de l'enseignement médical et au développement de la recherche médicale. 1958. *Journal Officiel,* December 31, 1958.

Organization for Economic Cooperation and Development. 1972. *The research system I: France, Germany, United Kingdom.* Paris.

————. 1974. *Study of education of the health professions in the context of health care systems.* Paris.

Peterson, H. 1975. The Stockholm County medical information system. In *Computer information systems in health care.* London: Sperry Univac.

Petit, J. 1976. *Verslag over de Ziekteverzekering.* Brussels: Kamer van Volksvertegenwoordigers.

Polack, J. C. 1971. *La médecine du capital.* Paris: Maspero.

President of the United States. 1976. *Message concerning the State of the Union.* Washington, D.C.: U.S. Government Printing Office, 94th Congress.

Pruvost, R., and Y. Samson. 1974. *La réforme hospitalière du 31 décembre 1970.* Rennes: Ecole nationale de la Santé Publique.

Querido, A. 1965. *Een eeuw staatstoezicht op de volksgezondheid.* The Hague: Staatsuitgeverij.

————. 1973. Medical education, care and research in the Netherlands. In *Medical research systems in Europe,* pp. 143–52. Amsterdam: Elsevier, Excerpta Medica.

Rachold, R. 1967. *Bestallungsordnung für Ärzte.* Cologne, Berlin: Deutsche Ärzte Verlag.

Raynaud, P. 1971. La loi hospitalière et les hôpitaux publics. *La Revue hospitalière de France* 35:163–88.

————. 1974. Mémorandum à Madame le Ministre de la Santé sur les établissements hospitaliers publics. *La Revue hospitalière de France* 38:929–47.

Rexed, B. 1971. Public policy and medicine. In *The Swedish health services system,* pp. 199–218. Chicago: ACHA.

————. 1974. The role of medical education in planning the development of a national health care system. *Journal of Medical Education* 49:27–42.

————. 1975. How Sweden plans for the 1980's. In *The health care cost explosion,* pp. 67–82. Bern: Hans Huber.

Riksförsäkringsverket. 1975. *Social security in Sweden.* Stockholm.

Rimlinger, G. V. 1971. *Welfare policy and industrialization in Europe, America and Prussia.* New York: John Wiley.

Robinson, K. 1968. *The administrative structure of the medical and related services in England and Wales (green paper 1).* London: HMSO.

Rösch, E. 1973. *Elements de économique médicale.* Paris: Flammarion.

Rosenthal, A. H. 1969. *The social programs of Sweden.* Minneapolis: University of Minnesota Press.

Royal Commission on the National Health Service, 1976. *The task of the commission.* London: HMSO.

Schadewaldt, H., P. P. Grzonka, and G. Lenz. 1975. *75 Jahre Hartmannbund.* Verband der Ärzte Deutschlands.

Schellenberg, E. 1968. *Von der Sozialversicherung zur Volksversicherung.* Munich: Institut für Sozialpolitik und Arbeitsrecht.

Schlauss, H. J. *Die Ausgabe der gesetzlichen Krankenversicherung für Krankenhauspflege im Jahrzehnt 1958 bis 1967.*

Sénat, A. 1973. Etudes analytiques à l'échelon national des effectifs des infirmières. *La Revue hospitalière de France* 37:567–80.

Servan-Schreiber, J. J. 1967. *Le défi américain.* Paris: Denoël.

Shenkin, B. 1973. Politics and medical care in Sweden: the seven crowns reform. *New England Journal of Medicine* 288:551–59.

———. 1974. Medical education, medical care and society in Sweden. *Journal of Medical Education* 49:357–67.

Siderius, P. 1975. European studies of drug consumption. In *The health care cost explosion,* pp. 139–48. Bern: Hans Huber.

Sigerist, H. E. 1960. *On the sociology of medicine.* New York: M. D. Publications.

Sijses, P. 1968. *Algemene Wet Bijzondere Ziektekosten.* Deventer: Kluwer.

Sociale verzekeringswetten, Deel 1, A.W.B.Z. Deventer: Kluwer.

Socialstyrelsen. 1973. *Hälso- och sjukvård inför ör 80-talet* Stockholm.

———. 1974. *Allman Halsö- och sjukvård 1972.* Stockholm: Sveriges Officiella Statistik.

Somers, H. 1972. National health insurance: strategy and standards. *Medical Care* 10:81–87.

Spiegel, Der. 1977 (31:8). Ärzte gegen Bonn.

Staatssekretaris Hendriks beantwoordt vragen rondom de Structuurnota Gezondheidszorg. 1975. *Medisch Contact* 30:701–7.

Steudler, F. 1974. *L'hôpital en observation.* Paris: Colin.

Stevens, R. 1966. *Medical practice in modern England.* New Haven: Yale University Press.

Stichting Medische Registratie. 1969. *Classificatie van ziekten voor de medische registratie in ziekenhuizen.* Lochem: De Tijdstroom.

Stump, W. 1973. Sozial politik im kaiserlichen Deutschland. *Viertal Jahresschrift für Sozialrecht* 1973:2–3.

Swedish Institute, The. 1974. *Local administration in Sweden.* Stockholm.

———. 1975. *The Swedish population.* Stockholm.

Swedish Medical Association. 1971. *Effects of the seven kronor reform.* Stockholm.

Swedish Planning and Rationalization Institute (SPRI). 1971. *Guidelines for public health planning, 14/71.* Stockholm.

———. 1972. *Den öppna vårdens organisation.* Stockholm.

———. 1974. *Documentation.* Stockholm.

Tengstam, A. 1975. *Patterns of health care and education in Sweden.* Paris: Organization for Economic Cooperation and Development.

Thapper, F. 1967. The regional plan. In *Regional hospital planning: in honour of A. Engel.* Stockholm: National Board of Health.

Titmuss, R. 1958. *Essays on the welfare state.* London: Allen and Unwin.

———. *Health.* London: Stevens.

Tomasson, R. F. 1970. *Sweden: prototype of modern society.* New York: Random House.

Van den Berg, C. 1965. Het staatstoezicht op de ziekenfondsen in het bevrijde zuiden van ons land. *Het Ziekenfonds* 1965:110–16.

————. 1965. De ziekenfondsen ten tijde van de bevrijding. *Het Ziekenfonds* 1965:133–38.

Van de Vijsel, A. 1977. Planning en budgetering in de N. H. S. *Medisch Contact* 32:173–77.

Van Es, J. C. 1968. *Maatschappelijke gezondheidszorg in perspectief.* Assen: Van Gorcum.

Van Langendonck, J. 1971. *De harmonisering van de sociale verzekering voor gezondheidszorgen in de E.E.G.* Leuven: Instituut voor Sociaal Zekerheidsrecht.

————. 1975. *Prelude to harmony on a community theme, health care insurance policies in the Six and Britain.* London: Oxford University Press for the Nuffield Provincial Hospitals Trust.

Veldkamp, G. M. J. 1967. Sociale zekerheid en gezondheidszorg. *Sociaal Maandblad Arbeid* 1967:6.

Verdoorn, J. 1972. *Arts en oorlog.* Amsterdam: Lynx.

Verduyn, J. 1966. Ontwerp wet algemene verzekering zware geneeskundige risico's. *Sociaal Maandblad Arbeid* 1966:342–43.

Verordnung zur Regelung der Krankenhauspflegesätze. 1973. *Bundesgesetzblatt* 1973:333.

Waldman, S. 1976. *National health insurance proposals.* Washington, D.C.: Department of Health, Education, and Welfare.

Watkin, B. 1975. *Documents on health and social services.* London: Methuen.

Wet van 14 december 1967 houdende Algemene Verzekering Bijzondere Ziektekosten. 1967. *Staatsblad van het Koninkrijk der Nederlanden* 1967:655.

Wet van 25 maart 1971 houdende regelen ter bevordering van doelmatige voorzieningen terzake van ziekenhuizen en andere inrichtingen voor gezondheidszorg. 1971. *Staatsblad von het Koninkrijk der Nederlanden* 1971:268.

Werkö, L. 1971. Swedish medical care in transition. *New England Journal of Medicine* 284:360–66.

Willcocks, A. 1967. *The creation of the national health service.* London: Routledge.

Wissenschaftsrat. 1965. *Empfehlungen des Wissenschaftrates zum Ausbau der wissenschaftlichen Einrichtungen.*

Working party on the education and training of senior managers in the N.H.S. 1977. *Invitation to initiative.* London: King's Fund.

World Health Organization. 1972. *Training in hospital administration in Europe.* Copenhagen.

Ziekenfondsraad. 1965. *25 jaar Ziekenfondswetgeving.*

Ziekenfondsenbesluit. 1941. *Staatsblad van het Koninkrijk der Nederlanden* 1941:804.

Index